Meat, vegetables, eggs...
This could be the
Over the Moon Farm diet!
—Amy

P9-BJW-763

END YOUR
CARB
CONFUSION

A Simple Guide to Customize
Your Carb Intake for Optimal Health

ERIC C. WESTMAN, MD

with AMY BERGER, CNS

Eric Westman

Amy Berger

VICTORY BELT PUBLISHING INC.
LAS VEGAS

First published in 2021 by Victory Belt Publishing Inc.

Copyright © 2021 Eric C. Westman and Amy Berger

All rights reserved

No part of this publication may be reproduced or distributed in any form or by any means, electronic or mechanical, or stored in a database or retrieval system, without prior written permission from the publisher.

ISBN-13: 978-1-628604-29-0

The information included in this book is for educational purposes only. It is not intended or implied to be a substitute for professional medical advice. The reader should always consult his or her healthcare provider to determine the appropriateness of the information for his or her own situation or if he or she has any questions regarding a medical condition or treatment plan. Reading the information in this book does not constitute a physician-patient relationship. The statements in this book have not been evaluated by the Food and Drug Administration. The products or supplements in this book are not intended to diagnose, treat, cure, or prevent any disease. The authors and publisher expressly disclaim responsibility for any adverse effects that may result from the use or application of the information contained in this book.

Illustrations by Jenny Gough Short and Crizalie Olimpo

Cover design by James Woolley

Interior design by Crizalie Olimpo

Printed in Canada

TC 0121

CONTENTS

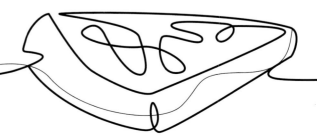

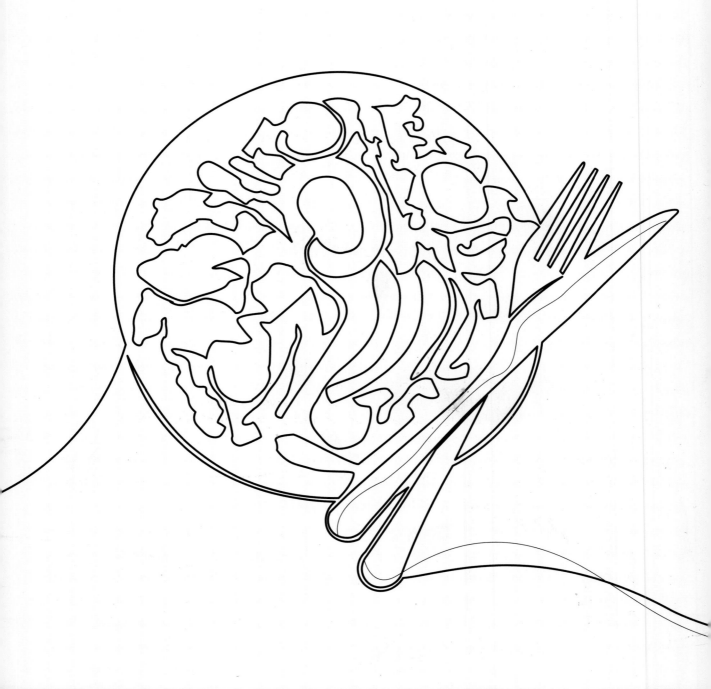

INTRODUCTION

Do you feel totally overwhelmed by the avalanche of information out there about diet and health? Have you given up even *trying* to figure out what's right for you? Low-carb? Low-fat? Vegetarian? Keto? Mediterranean? Or have you gone the opposite way, immersing yourself in everything you can get your eyes and ears on—every video and podcast, every book, blog, forum, social media feed, and program from self-proclaimed experts? Maybe not a second goes by that you're not scrolling through things on your phone or immersed in what's coming through your earbuds, and you still have no idea which way to go.

Maybe you already feel great, you're happy with what you see in the mirror, and you want to make sure you're doing the right things to keep this good thing you've got going long into the future. Or maybe you know something isn't right, and you've been trying to figure out how to help yourself. Either way, if you feel frustrated, confused, and maybe even a little angry, you're not alone.

Every day in my clinic, I see patients who are struggling. I talk with people whose quality of life is being shortchanged by excess weight, diabetes, heart disease, joint pain, infertility, fatigue, severe acid reflux, and a long list of other issues that plague so many adults these days—maybe even you. Some of these people grew up eating whatever they liked and carried those same habits into adulthood. They never paid much attention to the kinds of foods they ate, and now that they're older, things they "got away with" as kids are catching up to them. Others have spent years, sometimes decades, following advice they thought would result in optimal health and help them get to a weight they were happy with, only to end up feeling the three Ds—disappointed, disheartened, and discouraged—and often heavier and sicker than when they started.

I understand their frustration. It's especially maddening when you think you're doing all the right things. You devote time, effort, and often a lot of money into pursuing a strategy that "everyone knows" will work. If you're carrying excess weight, you've cut your calories and gotten yourself on a treadmill or elliptical machine most days of the week. If you have acid reflux, you've cut out tomato sauces, spicy foods, and maybe even your beloved coffee—everything the experts said to stop eating and drinking because they would aggravate the problem. If you have cardiovascular disease, you've probably done what many doctors and nutritionists advise without a second thought: ditched red meat, eggs, bacon, and butter in favor of salmon, walnuts, whole grains, fruit, and as many green vegetables as you can cram onto your plate.

But what has happened? If you feel better and your problems have been resolved, great! It's more likely, though, that your problems haven't been resolved. In fact, they might even be worse. But it's not your fault. Let me say that again: *it's not your fault.*

When you follow bad advice and get bad results, is the failure yours, or is the problem with the advice? To borrow a phrase I like, "It's not your fault, but it is your *responsibility*." However, you can be responsible for making effective choices only when you know what those effective choices are. If something doesn't work—especially if it hasn't worked over and over and over again, despite your best efforts—should you keep trying that same thing, only work harder at it? Or would it be smarter to step back and look at things from a different perspective? When you have better information, you can try a better strategy. This is where you take responsibility—or, more accurately, *you take control.* Why use an outdated paper map from 50 years ago that shows obsolete roads when you can use a GPS that's updated every minute? Better navigation means an easier journey to your destination, whether you're talking about your car or your body.

But what is the nutritional GPS? Which approach is the right one for you? Do you feel like a deer in headlights when you're faced with the mountains of books on nutrition and health? Do you go on buying sprees with your favorite online bookseller, read everything, and end up more confused than ever? Are there five, eight, ten, or *twenty* people you follow online, all of whom look like dynamite and appear to be in perfect health, but their ways of doing things are entirely different from each other?

It doesn't have to be this way. People weren't always so unwell and overwhelmed, and you don't need to feel that way now.

I'm going to share with you what I've learned in more than 20 years of helping people lose weight, reverse chronic illness, and recover their vitality and zest for life. The first and most important thing to know is that *this is simple.* I'm sometimes stunned at the size of diet and health books I see. Four hundred pages? How could it possibly be so complicated? And who has time to read all that, anyway? The people who come to my clinic have jobs, families, responsibilities, and commitments. They need something straightforward and *uncomplicated.*

Some people want the nitty-gritty details. They want to understand the science, such as the name of every molecule or the ins and outs of every biochemical pathway. But most people are happy to leave all that behind in high school biology class. What I hear most often from my patients is, "Just tell me what to do, Doc."

So I'm going to do that—with your help.

Whether you're looking to lose body fat, improve a health problem, or find a way of eating that you can stick with to sustain good health for the rest of your life without having to ping-pong between whatever new diet fad comes along every 30 seconds, let this book be your GPS to help you navigate toward the strategy that's right for you.

Keep in mind that GPS works only when you know where you're starting from and where you want to go—your current location and your destination. This is where you come in: You know your body best, just as you know your car. You know where you've been, the bumps and potholes you've gone over through the years, and the dings and dents you've accumulated. It's okay if you've collected a few scratches and rust spots along the way; none of us is in perfect factory condition. But together, we'll get you as close to shiny, new, and revving to go as you can be. You don't need a brand-new engine; maybe all you need to do is change the fuel you're using.

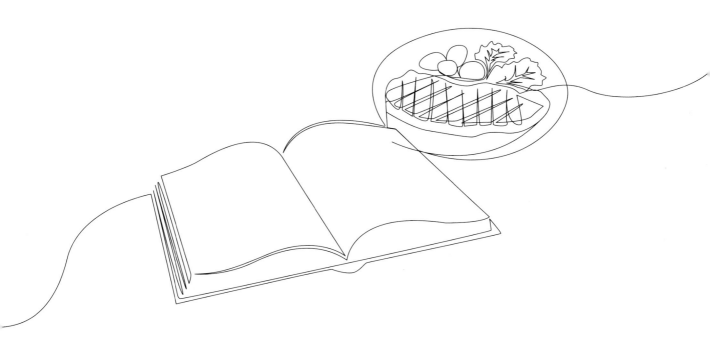

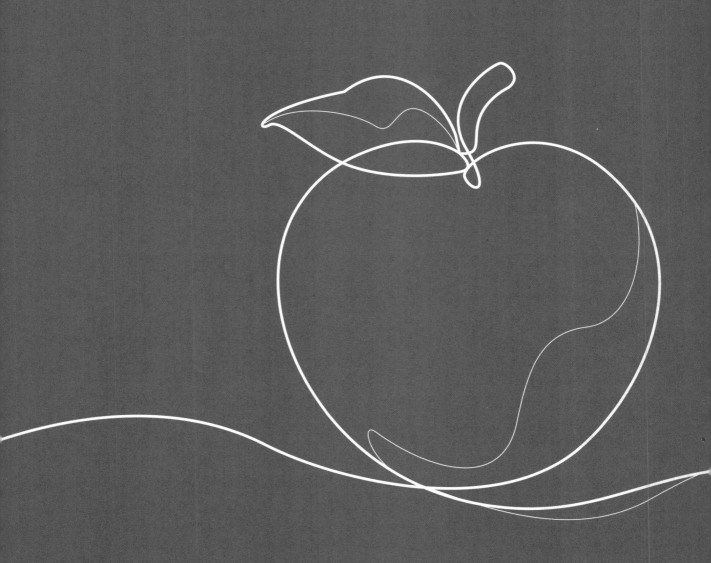

HOW WE GOT HERE

CHAPTER 1

WHY THE CURRENT APPROACH TO DIET AND HEALTH IS FAILING

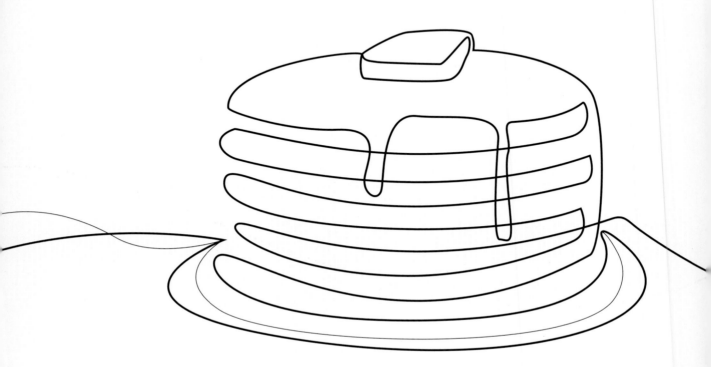

It's not hard to see the crisis. Take a look around. It's impossible to ignore that people aren't as healthy as they could be. If you do some people-watching at an airport, at a shopping center, or in a coffee shop, there's no denying that epidemics of obesity, type 2 diabetes, chronic pain and fatigue, mental health disturbances, and a slew of other issues are robbing people of quality and quantity of life. People are dying younger, and the years they do live often aren't as enjoyable as they could be because they carry extra weight, have aching joints, and deal with chronic indigestion, acid reflux, skin problems, infertility, anxiety, depression, sleep issues, and a seemingly endless list of other ailments.

Robbing isn't the right word, though. Unlike a thief who comes in the night, takes all your valuables, and changes your life quite literally overnight, the health problems many people face these days come on slowly. They happen over years. You don't gain 40, 50, or 100 extra pounds in a week or even a few months. Your blood sugar doesn't get out of control after just one chocolate milkshake or a mammoth stack of pancakes with syrup at your favorite breakfast spot. These things take years—sometimes decades—to develop. And what's worse is they come on so slowly that you don't even notice they're happening until they're already out of control.

How did we get here?

The Fear of Dietary Fat Led to Obesity and Type 2 Diabetes Epidemics

Let's cut right to the chase: The very foods you've been advised to eat for decades—foods that are low in fat and high in carbohydrates—set you up to feel hungry and irritable all day. You don't feel satiated because these foods don't give you the protein and fat you need to feel full and satisfied for several hours. And when you give in to your hunger—to this very natural, biologically normal drive to eat—you feel like a failure. Your doctor or nutritionist told you to eat less, and you can't seem to do that because you're so darn hungry all the time.

I said it in the introduction, and I'll repeat it: You're not alone. There are people whose entire lives revolve around food. During breakfast, they think about what they'll have for lunch. At lunch, they wonder what's for dinner, and in between, there are snacks and invasive thoughts of food all day long. Is this abnormal, or is it exactly how you should expect to feel when you're following advice that keeps you trapped in an endless cycle of hunger? When satellites fail, signals are lost, and the GPS is offline, you lose your way and drive around in circles.

For the last few decades, it's been recommended that people get the majority of calories from carbohydrates. Who could forget that iconic food pyramid, with bread, pasta, rice, cereal, and other starches and grains at the base? However, only two generations ago, people judged the quality of milk by the thick layer of rich cream at the top, and back then, obesity, type 2 diabetes, and most of the other health problems people face today were rare.

Our grandparents would laugh at the notion of getting on a treadmill and running to nowhere or climbing a set of fake stairs. Sure, if your grandparents or great-grandparents were farmers or laborers, they got a lot of exercise every day without even trying. Physical activity was a natural part of their everyday lives. But if you look at pictures of commuters on buses and trains on their way to work in urban areas in the 1950s and 1960s, overweight and obese people were rare in those settings, too. So just a few decades ago, even people who had sedentary jobs were mostly lean, and the incidence of type 2 diabetes and other metabolic diseases was low.

And what are we supposed to make of toddlers with obesity? I'm not talking about infants being a bit pudgy, the way they're supposed to be. I'm talking about genuine obesity in toddlers and adolescents—excess weight to the point that their health is jeopardized. Children are also being diagnosed with fatty liver—a condition once reserved solely for adults, and more precisely, for adults who drank a lot of alcohol. Now it's called nonalcoholic fatty liver disease because it occurs even in adults who steer clear of booze—and in children.

What's going on here? When a toddler or young child has obesity, type 2 diabetes, a fatty liver, or another severe health issue, is it all the child's fault? Should they have simply eaten less and moved more in the womb? We need to come up with a better explanation than that these toddlers aren't exercising enough. Something else is behind these problems; young children shouldn't have to count calories, and neither should you.

Eat Less, Move More?

If you've struggled to lose weight over the years, you're no doubt intimately familiar with the following four words: *eat less, move more*. On the surface, this sounds like perfectly logical advice. If you take in less energy than your body uses, then something has to make up for that shortage, right? And where else would that come from but your stored body fat?

It sounds reasonable. Too bad it doesn't work in practice, though. Math is for calculators and computers, not for the human body, and the concept of calories is misleading. A calorie is a unit of measure; it describes how much energy is stored in a food and how much energy you would get from metabolizing it—that is, from breaking it down to give your cells energy. The problem is that calories were calculated using a device called a *bomb calorimeter*. Think of it as a box with insides that have no interaction with the outside world. After you put food in the box, the box is sealed up, and the food is burned until there's nothing left. It gets completely broken down.

That's called a *closed system*, and it works well for physics experiments. However, the human body is not a closed system. If someone's ever tried to explain calorie counting to you and invoked "eat less, move more" by talking about the laws of thermodynamics, they misunderstand a fundamental premise: the first law of thermodynamics applies only to closed systems.

Unlike a closed system, your body is an open system because you interact with the environment. You breathe, sweat, urinate, defecate, and pass gas. You lose heat, water, and gases like carbon dioxide. Right here, you can see that the concept of calories is less helpful than it seems.

The second flaw in the calorie concept relates to what I mentioned earlier about calories being units of measure. Think about a pound, which is also a unit of measure. (Calories measure energy and pounds measure weight, just like miles and kilometers measure distance, and cups and liters measure liquid volume.) In the same way that a calorie is a calorie, a pound is a pound. One hundred calories of avocado contain the same energy as one hundred calories of honey because, indeed, a calorie is a calorie. Just like a thousand pounds of bricks weighs the same as a thousand pounds of feathers, because a pound is a pound. When you're building a house, though, there's a huge difference between a thousand pounds of bricks and a thousand pounds of feathers. One is very useful to you; the other is a total waste of space. A pound is a pound, but *what those pounds consist of and what you can use them for are entirely different.*

To bring this discussion back to calories, the biochemical and hormonal effects of different kinds of calories are entirely different. It's irrelevant that 100 calories of avocado and 100 calories of honey provide equal numbers of calories. Your body doesn't deal in calories; it deals in hormones, enzymes, and metabolic processes with feedback loops that rival the blueprints for building the International Space Station. It's not that calories are meaningless, but when you're looking to control your appetite, lose weight, and get your health back, what your body does with calories is far more important than the number of calories you consume.

Let's tackle this calorie thing from an even more interesting angle. Even knowing that the concept of calories is highly flawed when applied to the human body, let's proceed using the general rule that fat provides 9 calories per gram, and carbohydrates and protein both provide 4 calories per gram. So 1 gram of fat gives you more than double the calories of 1 gram of carbohydrate or protein. With this in mind, if you need to consume fewer calories to lose weight, it makes sense to limit high-fat foods and fill up on protein and carbs. Eating more protein in this context is difficult because unless you stick to canned tuna, skinless chicken breast, egg whites, and protein shakes, most protein comes naturally packaged with fat—like a steak, pork chop, chicken leg, or salmon fillet. Because these protein-rich foods also can be high in fat, and therefore high in calories, carbs seem like a better way to go when you're trying to eat fewer calories. And if you really want to kick fat loss into high gear, eating a low-fat, high-carb diet and doing a lot of exercise should be a slam dunk. Unfortunately, this works much better on paper than it works in people.

> If you want to **kick fat loss** into high gear, eating a **low-fat**, **high-carb diet** and doing a lot of exercise should be a slam dunk. Unfortunately, **this works much better on paper** than it works in people.

"Eat less, move more" sounds so logical that it became enshrined as the go-to advice for anyone carrying extra weight. But this advice ignores basic biology. It's like putting less gas in your car and expecting to drive farther. It doesn't work on the road, and it doesn't work so well in your body, either.

If you put less gas in your tank but then try to cover more distance, eventually your tank will be empty, and you'll be stranded on the side of the road, going nowhere. Your body is smarter than that; it will compensate for the reduced amount of energy coming in and the increase in energy being expended. If you were to move more, and then move more and more and more, while continually giving yourself less fuel (eat less, move more), you'd run out of gas and stall out. To prevent this from happening—to protect you—your body slows down your metabolism. It compensates for the reduced amount of energy coming in to keep you from burning out.

You're probably accustomed to thinking about "burning calories" through deliberate physical activity—things like walking, running, swimming, biking, weightlifting, and other forms of exercise. But your body burns energy all day long, even while you're sleeping. Your body uses most of the energy it generates just to keep you alive. (You might have heard this referred to as your *basal metabolic rate*.) Your cells use an enormous amount of energy in processes you can't even see, but which, in total, use far more energy than you would reasonably expend even in a long and intense workout. When you force your body to perform activities for which you're not adequately fueling it, your body slows things down to keep you from running out of gas. You start to use less energy for those invisible cellular processes, and your metabolic rate will be set to low.

When this happens, the amount of food that used to be enough to keep your weight constant or allow you to lose weight becomes too much. Operating under the calorie paradigm, you'd have to eat even less to continue to lose weight. Unfortunately, your metabolic rate is slower, so eating less to lose weight doesn't work, and you assume you have to exercise more, too. This awful cycle keeps going until you either burn out physically and emotionally or give up in well-earned frustration and find yourself facedown in a large pizza with the works. So much for the "eat less, move more" approach.

Hunger

Flaws in the calorie concept aren't the biggest problem with the advice to base your diet on starchy carbohydrates and keep fat intake low. The real issue is *hunger!* Whether your goal is to lose weight, improve your blood sugar, lower your blood pressure, or address some other issue, you are not going to stick with a way of eating that keeps you hungry. *No one* can.

Asking you to adhere long term to a diet that leaves you hungry all the time is like telling you to ignore the urge to breathe and simply not take in a breath when you need one. It might work for a short time—a few seconds in the case of breathing, maybe a few weeks or months in the case of food—but eventually biology will win out, and you *will* take a breath or satisfy your hunger. You *will* dive headfirst into the bag of chips, the box of cookies, the tub of frosting, or whatever it is you've been trying to pretend doesn't exist. You can resist a physical drive that is biologically hardwired into you for only so long. And guess what? *You shouldn't have to.*

The issue isn't about willpower or discipline. You can hold your breath for a few seconds, and some people have trained themselves to go a few *minutes*, but no amount of willpower can keep you from taking a breath when you really, really need one. And no amount of discipline can keep you from eating when your body and brain are screaming for food. You can fight hunger for a while, but biology eventually will win. Every time. Don't feel bad for losing to your hardwiring; it had a head start of a few million years on you.

> " *Eat less, move more* sounds so logical that it became **enshrined as the go-to advice** for anyone carrying extra weight. But this advice **ignores basic biology**. It's like **putting less gas in your car** and expecting to **drive farther**. It doesn't work on the road, and **it doesn't work so well in your body**, either.

Instead of fighting biology, what if you could work with it? Use it to your advantage? What if there were a way of eating that *didn't* leave you hungry all the time? What if you didn't have to white-knuckle your way through every meal, every dinner out, every social occasion?

There is, and the ADAPT Your Life Diet will show you the version of it that's right for you. You're going to call a truce with your biology—shake its hand and agree to work together instead of bashing your head against it and coming away mangled and bruised every time. You have an alternative: a way of eating that controls hunger and cravings, so you don't have to fight them. You don't have to will yourself to resist cravings when the cravings aren't there. The ADAPT Your Life Diet will show you how.

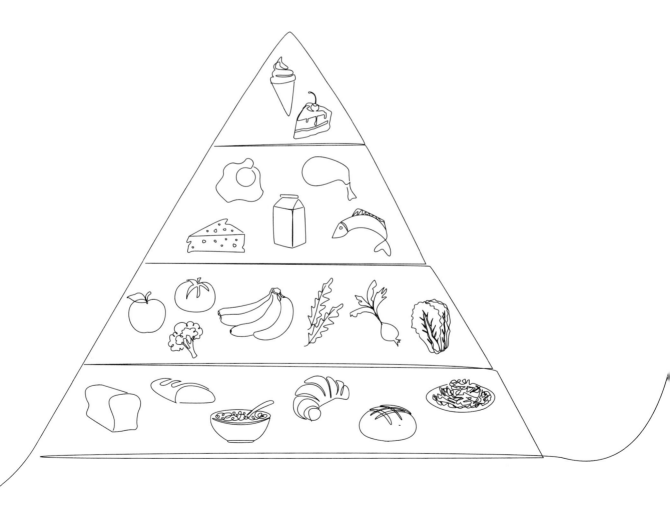

CHAPTER 2

SUGAR: ROBBER, WRECKER, WRESTLER

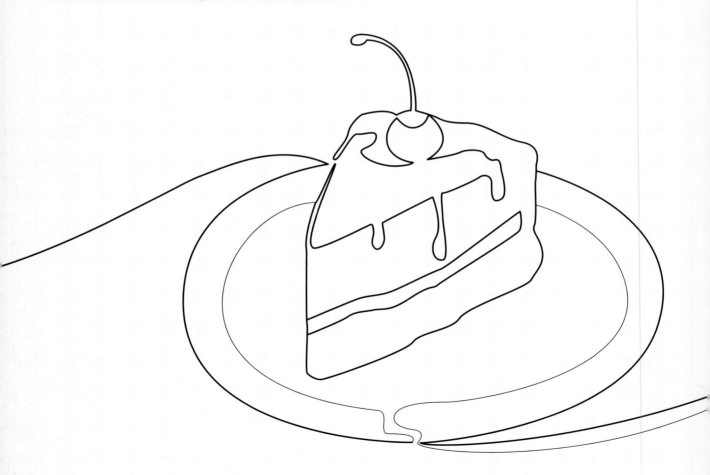

Why do so many people feel perpetually hungry on high-carb diets? It has a lot more to do with hormones than it does with calories.

When you eat carbohydrates, your blood sugar rises. Certain types of carbs have a more significant effect on blood sugar than others, but as a general rule, carbs affect blood sugar more than protein and fat do. In response to rising blood sugar, your pancreas secretes insulin, a hormone that helps bring blood sugar back down. (Insulin does a lot more than this, though—more on that in the next chapter.) In some people, this system works perfectly. Their bodies produce just the right amount of insulin to return their blood sugar to normal within a short time after eating. In others, however, the pancreas gets a bit aggressive. It secretes a large amount of insulin in response to carbs—refined carbs in particular—which ends up overshooting and bringing blood sugar down too low, resulting in low blood sugar. Other people have a different problem: their pancreas secretes a large amount of insulin, but their blood sugar stays high anyway.

There isn't an official definition for refined carbs. You can think of them as sugars and starches that have been removed from the foods they naturally occur in and are added in concentrated form to other foods, or sugars that have been manipulated so that your body absorbs them more quickly. The refining typically also removes the fiber, water, vitamins, and minerals that come naturally packaged with carbohydrate-dense foods, so when you eat refined carbs, your body gets the hit of carbohydrate minus these other nutrients that are provided in whole foods. For example, sugar crystals are refined carbs, as is high-fructose corn syrup. Bagels, pasta, cookies, crackers, toaster pastries, muffins, pita, tortilla chips, and breakfast cereal are examples of refined carbs, even if they're made with whole grains. Read more about this in Chapter 4.

If you've ever felt *hangry*—the combination of hungry and angry—that's low blood sugar, also called *hypoglycemia*. You feel irritable and anxious, your heart races, and you might even feel dizzy, nauseated, or confused. Most of all, you feel *hungry!* It's a feeling of panic, too—a sense of emergency when you don't find something to eat, *stat!* If you've ever felt this way, understand that there's nothing wrong with you. The problem isn't your body; the problem is the food you're eating.

People who are sensitive to carbohydrates in this way find it almost impossible to skip a meal or go without snacking between meals. A well-meaning doctor or dietitian might even recommend that a person snack throughout the day or have several small meals to "keep their blood sugar up." This advice is the exact opposite of what would help the person the most because it just perpetuates the problem. Snacking every couple of hours helps address the symptoms in the short term. If blood sugar dips too low, then yes, eating—eating carbs, especially—will bring it back up quickly. But why not address the root cause, so you don't get low blood sugar in the first place?

> If you've ever felt **hangry**—the combination of hungry and angry— that's **low blood sugar**. You feel **irritable, shaky, anxious,** and **hungry**! It's a feeling of panic, too—a sense of emergency when you don't find something to eat, *stat!* If you've ever felt this way, understand that there's nothing wrong with you. *The problem isn't your body; **the problem** is the food you're **eating**.*

If your blood sugar drops too low because of the flood of insulin after a high-carb meal or snack, why not just stop eating those carbs? Think of it like this: If your kitchen sink is overflowing because the drain is clogged, does it make sense to keep the faucet on full blast, get a bucket, and try to take water out faster than it's coming in, or would it be better to shut off the tap and *unclog the drain*? You can manage a crisis in the moment by dealing with the acute situation, but if you actually want to *fix the problem*, you have to address the cause. Get yourself off the blood sugar roller coaster by not getting on it in the first place.

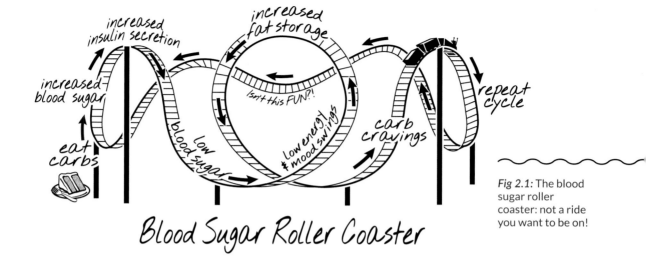

Blood Sugar Roller Coaster

Fig 2.1: The blood sugar roller coaster: not a ride you want to be on!

The Robber: Sugar Robs Nutrients

Sugar's list of offenses isn't limited to keeping you ping-ponging in hunger, energy levels, mood, and mental clarity all day. Those reasons alone would be enough to make most people think twice before eating high-sugar foods, but, the truth is, it's much worse than that. People use the phrase "empty calories" to point out that, with regard to nutrients—vitamins, minerals, amino acids, essential fats—sugar is a big ol' zero. It's a source of energy, but that's it. Calories with no redeeming nutrition. Zip. Zilch. But it's actually worse. Sugar *steals* nutrients from your body.

For your body to metabolize foods—to break them down and convert them to energy—you need several vitamins and minerals. The biochemical reactions involved don't happen by magic; they require things like magnesium, zinc, and B vitamins, but sugar brings none of these to the party. It shows up empty-handed, wreaks havoc, and then sneaks out with a prized family heirloom. Not a guest you want to invite back!

In terms of your health, when you eat refined sugar, it doesn't give you any of the vitamins or minerals your body requires to use it. So sugar doesn't just provide calories with no nutrients; it *increases your need* for nutrients so that your body has to get them from somewhere else—either from other foods you're consuming or from your body's stores. These nutrient shortfalls could be exacerbating some of the health issues you face now. You might not be deficient to the point of causing an overt deficiency disease (remember scurvy from high school health class—the sailors who had bleeding gums?), but you could be low enough in a critical nutrient that it's harming your health or making an existing problem worse. It's often said—correctly so—that in the modern era, people are *overfed but undernourished* because there's more than enough food to go around, but it's not all nutritious. More than enough calories, but not enough nutrients.

Naturally sweet or starchy whole foods that do provide nutrients along with their carbohydrates are a bit different. Things like sweet potatoes, beets, lentils, carrots, butternut squash, and black beans, for example, come with at least some of what your body needs to metabolize the foods and for overall health. Even so, if you have a significant health problem or are carrying a lot of excess body fat, even these natural, unrefined sweet or starchy foods may be too high in carbohydrate for you to include in your diet, at least at first. (Chapter 4 includes more about this.)

The Wrecker: Sugar Wrecks Health

Not long ago, many people in the medical and nutrition professions thought giving people cavities was the worst consequence of overeating sugar. We now know that cavities are a walk in the park (or maybe a trip to the dentist's office) compared to the other problems that result from consuming excessive sugar. Wrecking your teeth is only the beginning of the havoc sugar wreaks. There are no organs or tissues in the body that excessive sugar intake doesn't negatively impact. *None.* If you're living with type 2 diabetes or you've watched a loved one suffer the ravages of this disease, then you know the destruction chronically high blood sugar leaves in its wake. It affects the liver, kidneys, eyes, heart and blood vessels, brain, nerves, skin, and even the prostate, penis, and ovaries. Nothing is spared.

How do you know if you have chronically high blood sugar? Having your blood sugar—more formally called blood *glucose*—measured is a part of standard blood-work at a medical checkup. It's typically measured in a fasted state—you go to the lab or your doctor's office in the morning and have your blood drawn before you've had anything to eat or drink except water. This is your *fasting* glucose, which is a helpful measurement, but it has some shortcomings.

For starters, fasting glucose can be slightly elevated for several reasons, some of which could give you and your doctor the false impression that you're less healthy than you really are. For example, if you get stuck in a traffic jam on the way to the lab or deal with some other stressful situation before having your blood sample taken, your blood glucose will probably be a little higher than it otherwise would be. If it's just a bit higher than normal, it might not be cause for concern at all. If it's very high, though, then you and your doctor can look at other aspects of your bloodwork to see if a more serious issue is present.

> We used to think the **worst thing excess sugar** did was cause **cavities**. We now know that's among the least of the problems that come from **consuming too much sugar**.

However, even a normal fasting glucose level doesn't automatically mean you're in the clear concerning blood sugar control and metabolic health. Many people have normal fasting glucose, but when they eat a meal—especially a meal high in carbs—their blood glucose rises a lot and stays elevated for several hours. In some people, it doesn't come back down to normal before they're reaching for a snack or having their next meal, which means it's about to rise even more. This pattern keeps blood sugar high most of the day, even if the fasting level measured at a lab or doctor's office is normal. There's a different test that can fill in a little more of the picture here, called hemoglobin A1c, or A1c for short. Let's take a look at it.

Understanding the concept of glycation will help you make the connection between elevated blood sugar and the health problems you or someone you know may be afflicted with. There's a reason the word *glycation* sounds vaguely similar to *glucose*. Glycation is a process by which physical structures in your body—the proteins and fats that make up your cells, organs, tissues, and glands—become sticky with sugar. Imagine the way a piece of hard candy or a lollipop coats everything in a thick, sticky mess if it's left out on a hot summer day. Now, think of this happening to your blood, blood vessels, muscles, and other tissues, and you'll have some idea of what glycation is.

Glycated proteins—proteins that are mucked up with sugar—don't function properly. And when the proteins in your body don't function properly, *you* don't function properly. If you have diabetes, your doctor likely orders a hemoglobin A1c test for you at every visit, and you've probably had this measured a few times even if you don't have diabetes. The A1c test goes beyond your fasting glucose level. A1c measures glycated hemoglobin, which is the percentage of the hemoglobin protein in your blood that's become sticky with sugar. A1c is an indicator of what your average blood sugar level has been over the previous three months or so. It's a bit more complex than this, but as a general rule, the higher your A1c, the higher your blood sugar has been.

It's not just your blood that gets glycated, though. The vessels that carry your blood also are susceptible to glycation, which is why people with diabetes experience so many problems with their eyes and their kidneys. The eyes and kidneys contain tiny blood vessels that are very fragile and easily damaged from exposure to too much sugar in the blood. Diabetes is the number one cause of adult blindness and kidney failure in the United States. (The blood vessels in the eyes are so strongly affected by high blood sugar that an ophthalmologist is sometimes the first doctor to detect a patient's diabetes—and they don't even need a blood test to do it. While examining a patient's retinas, these doctors can see the damage that's already been caused.) Even the larger and hardier blood vessels, like arteries, take a beating from chronically high blood sugar. Cardiovascular disease—problems with the heart muscle and blood vessels—is the leading cause of death in people with type 2 diabetes. It's not because of fat or cholesterol in their diet; it's because of the sugar.

The nerve damage, or *neuropathy*, many people with diabetes experience is another consequence of glycated blood vessels. Blood vessels damaged from high blood sugar don't deliver blood as well as they should to the tissues they're responsible for. The farther these vessels are from the heart, the more affected they tend to be, which is why the pain, tingling, or numbness neuropathy causes is usually worst in the feet.

You might be surprised to learn that chronically high blood sugar is connected to erectile dysfunction (ED). That's right, guys. If you're dealing with this issue, then you know it's neither a libido problem nor because of a lack of attraction to your partner. You can't sustain an erection because the blood vessels supplying blood to your penis aren't working properly, and you can't get or maintain an erection without a boost of blood flow there. ED is a cardiovascular problem—one that might tip you off to the fact that your blood vessels are starting to suffer damage from constantly high blood sugar long before things get bad enough to progress to full-blown cardiovascular disease or type 2 diabetes. This is especially true for younger men, who should have no problems in this area. If you're a young guy with unexplained ED (meaning, you can't think of a reason why it's happening, such as depression or physical trauma to the area), take it seriously. It's an early warning sign that your blood sugar is too high, too often. The good news is, it's easily fixable. The ADAPT Your Life Diet will show you how.

People who experience migraines may be especially sensitive to rapid fluctuations in blood sugar. Many things can cause migraines in susceptible individuals, such as changes in barometric pressure or sensitivities to various scents (perfume, candles) and environmental compounds. Volatile ups and downs in blood sugar can be included in the list. Mood disorders are another category of problems linked to unstable blood sugar. As is true for migraines, there are numerous causes of anxiety, but wild swings in blood sugar play a big role for some people. Hypoglycemia, in particular, can trigger feelings of rage or panic. If you deal with hypoglycemia, you might even have family members who know you have these spells and who—if they're brave enough to approach at the moment of impact—suggest you have a candy bar or a glass of juice because they know the sugar will help calm you. Of course, the problem isn't a candy bar or juice deficiency right then; your blood sugar is tanking because of the high-carb food or drink you had earlier.

The Wrestler: Sugar Wrestles for Control

What if you're happy with your weight and don't have health concerns? Sugar can still be a problem. Sugar addiction is a real thing; don't let anyone tell you otherwise. If your physical health is fine, but you feel like a slave to sugar, then the addiction is compromising your mental and emotional health. Perhaps you take a detour to the donut shop on the way to or from work. Maybe you have candy wrappers peppering the floor of your car or a secret stash of sugary snacks hidden from your significant other or your kids, so no one sees the amount of junk you're eating. If you feel ashamed of your sugar habit and you feel out of control, getting this monkey off your back is absolutely a legitimate reason to follow a no-sugar diet.

It's a rare person who can eat five jelly beans or two cookies and then close the bag and forget about it for the rest of the day. Many people lose control around sugar. There's no off switch. If you have a weakness when you're around sugar and can't stop once you start, congratulations, you're human! No one can stop at just one.

> If you have a **weakness** when you're **around sugar** and can't stop once you start, congratulations, **you're human**! No one can **stop at just one**.

Sugary foods are designed to be addictive. They're *engineered* to be addictive. Entire industries are dedicated to studying the flavor and texture profiles that make people come back for more and more and more. Food manufacturers know biology and physiology better than some doctors do, and they use it to hijack your appetite. Sugar is even harder to resist when it's combined with fat—and even more so when flavoring is added. You wouldn't eat 7 teaspoons of white table sugar straight-up, but you probably have no problem eating that much when it's disguised in ice cream, caramel candies, cereal, or a milkshake. And you probably wouldn't eat sugar if it were mixed with only oil or butter, but add some flour, eggs, and cocoa powder, and you find the resulting chocolate cupcakes or brownies to be irresistible.

Irresistible, that is, *when you eat them.*

Sugar makes you wrestle with yourself. Your mind twists itself into knots trying to outsmart your opponent and engages in all kinds of tricks and maneuvers to stay one step ahead of sugar. Your inner monologue probably goes something like, "Should I eat it? Should I not eat it? I'll drink a glass of water to get my mind off it. I'll brush my teeth; I won't want to mess up a clean mouth. Maybe I'll have just one. I can't have just one, and I know it. No, this time will be different." Spoiler alert: *it's never different.*

Boxing is a good analogy, too. Sugar is a formidable opponent, and it will never let you win. So why not give up the fight? Walk out of the ring. You don't have to keep jabbing at it while it's preparing to land a huge right hook upside your head. Take yourself out of the match with your head—and your health—intact.

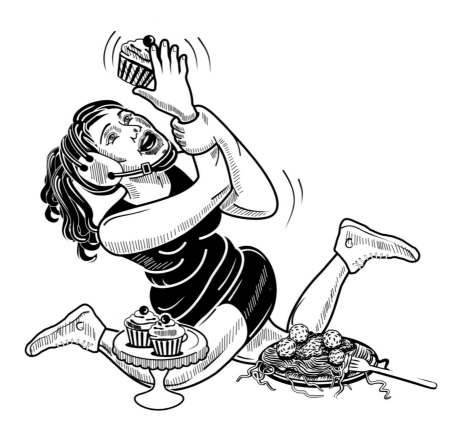

Fig 2.2: Want to win the wrestling match with sugar? Don't even step into the ring!

I said that sugar is irresistible when you eat it. *When you eat it* is the important point here. You crave what you eat. Eating sugar makes you want more sugar. Feeding the sugar beast doesn't satisfy it and make it go away; it makes it hungrier for more. You're probably used to hearing this piece of advice when it comes to cravings—maybe even from the little voice in your head: "Just eat it. Get it out of your system so you won't want it anymore." But how many times has this worked for you? Probably not many. When you give in to a sugar craving, you don't get it out of your system; you keep the cycle going. Sure, you've satisfied the urge at that moment, and five minutes later, you don't want any more, but a couple of hours later? The next day, the next week? You're thinking about that food again. And again and again.

Step out of that boxing ring and don't participate in the fight. When you stop feeding the beast, eventually it will stop asking to be fed. As I said, you don't need willpower to resist cravings when the cravings *aren't there*.

I know a life without sugar sounds mythical. Can you really have a day that isn't ruled by cravings—either giving in and feeling remorse and regret, or managing to resist but then feeling exhausted from spending all your energy fighting your own body and brain? Yes, it can be done. I see patients do it every day, and the feedback they give me most often is that it was much easier than they thought it would be. You can show sugar who's boss and get it out of your life. The ADAPT Your Life Diet will teach you how. Chapter 6 will help you determine which phase is right for you.

> " You **crave** what you **eat**. Eating sugar makes you **want more sugar**. Feeding the sugar beast doesn't **satisfy** it and make it **go away**; it makes it **hungrier for more**.

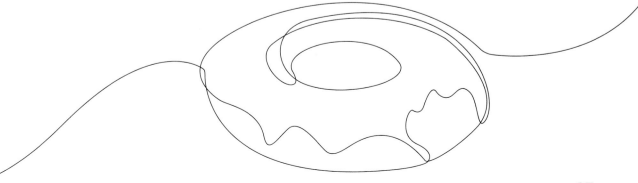

Binge Eating, Autoimmune Conditions, and Piles of Pills to Being in Control and Medication-Free

"I felt that the compulsion to binge and starve was gone."

My battle began early on when I was around nine or ten years old. I know now that I was never really overweight, and certainly not obese, but after being bullied pretty badly in fourth grade, I knew I looked different. I was bigger than everyone else. Yes, in my young mind, everyone. A comment made by a classmate in fifth grade confirmed it: I was "fat." I vowed from that point on, I would do whatever it took to be "skinny," like everyone else.

Throughout the following eight years, I dieted the best a child could. I copied what my friends ate, thinking, "If I eat what they do, I will look like them." As a multisport athlete in high school, I was in great shape, but that wasn't good enough for me. I was bigger. Over-the-counter diet pills and running 75 to 100 miles per week was my normal. I was still bigger.

One would think that once my brain finished developing and I became an adult, these silly practices would end. To the contrary, they got worse. As a working adult, I had access to more resources! The internet was becoming more prevalent. I was still taking every over-the-counter diet pill available, but now I was able to seek out international online pharmacies to lie to and order prescription diet pills from. Exciting times for me. What exactly these "pharmacies" sent me, I have no idea. I honestly didn't care. I took them anyway. I tried every commercial diet available at one time or another. They never worked, and I never stuck with any of them.

Bingeing and starving was a way of life for me. For more than 25 years, I binged for weeks to months at a time, followed by periods of up to 3 weeks with no food whatsoever. A single day of binge eating for me would start on my way to work: stopping at the donut shop for a bagel with cream cheese (low-fat, of course) and a bacon, egg, and cheese bagel. I would eat those in the 8 minutes it took to get to the fast food chain nearby. There, I would order two bacon, egg, and cheese biscuits and two egg muffins. I would eat those during the rest of my drive, stopping only to throw the wrappers in a trash barrel along the way, for fear they would be discovered in my car. At work, I had a salad every time I ate lunch with clients or colleagues. As far as anyone knew, I only ate salads with low-fat dressing.

Once home for the evening, the binge continued until every scrap of food in the house was gone. At that point, I would make boxed cake or brownie mixes and eat the entire bowl of batter. The compulsion to eat was so strong that sleep eluded me for days on end; I was making runs to fast food restaurants and grocery stores in the middle of the night regularly, and I always hid the wrappers underneath other household trash. I ate until the point of vomiting. I ate foods I didn't even like. I just ate. Everything. I had to.

When the guilt, shame, and pure self-loathing finally got the best of me, I would consume no food for up to three weeks at a time. Then it was time to binge again. This cycle continued for more than twenty-five years.

In my mid-thirties, I began to get sick. Very sick. After a year of testing and working with a team of nine different doctors, I was diagnosed with five confirmed autoimmune diseases: lupus, Epstein-Barr virus, Sjögren's syndrome, Raynaud's syndrome, and arthritis. Fibromyalgia was thrown in just for fun. Twenty-four daily prescription medications kept my flare-ups to approximately three to four per year. Flare-ups, of course, required an added regimen of prednisone—which causes weight gain and does nothing to help a weight problem or body dysmorphia.

I was still dieting and suffering through painful workouts, and I moved to a new city and got a new neighbor. While visiting one afternoon, my new neighbor mentioned that she didn't eat sugar or wheat and ate a low-carbohydrate, high-fat diet. "Atkins!" I proclaimed. "I've done that." "No," she said, "This is not Atkins." As she began telling me about the ketogenic diet and why she chose to eat this way, all I could think was, "Here's the one diet I haven't tried! I'm in!" I wish I could say that I started the ketogenic diet for the right reasons. I didn't. I stayed on keto for the right reasons. Four-and-a-half years later, the excess 25 pounds (11 kg) are still gone, and I haven't taken a single medication or had an autoimmune flare-up in more than four years. Today, I am still at a healthy weight, and I'm free of medications and autoimmune symptoms. The migraine headaches that plagued me for decades ended more than three years ago. I felt that the compulsion to binge and starve was gone.

Finding your best ketogenic diet takes time. Through much self-experimentation, I have found that, for me, maintaining a strict diet serves my health best. Tracking my food intake helps me maintain control over my binge eating and allows me to live life to the fullest.

—Robyn D., Long Beach, MS

CHAPTER 3

INSULIN: MORE THAN A BLOOD SUGAR HORMONE

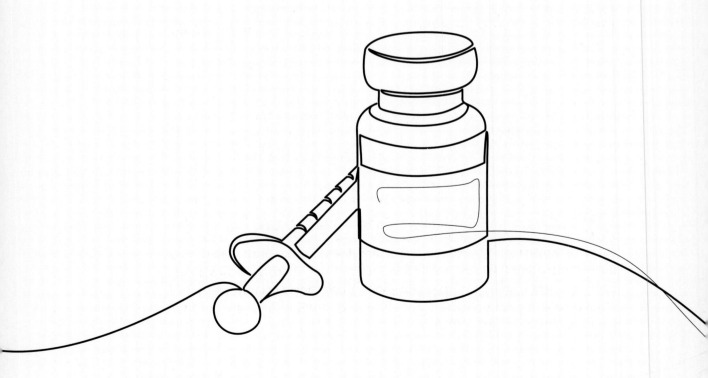

In Chapter 2, I talked a lot about blood sugar and the negative effects of blood sugar that's too high, too often. However, another problem—a much bigger one, in fact—is lurking in the shadows of high blood sugar: high insulin. I explained that having a normal fasting blood sugar level doesn't automatically mean you're free of cardiometabolic problems or that your body tolerates sugar well. Hemoglobin A1c provides a little more information in this area: if your fasting glucose is normal, but your A1c is high, then you know your blood sugar is often elevated, even if it comes back down to normal after several hours without food, such as when you wake up in the morning or when you fast for a blood test.

Just like fasting glucose, though, A1c has a shortcoming and doesn't always tell you the full story about your blood sugar. Many people—millions, in fact—have normal fasting glucose and normal A1c, but these measurements are normal because they're being kept in check by chronically elevated insulin. Elevated insulin is a major culprit behind health and weight struggles *even when blood sugar is normal.*

> **Elevated insulin** is a **major culprit** behind health and weight struggles *even when **blood sugar is normal**.*

Think for a minute about hormones other than insulin. Very few hormones have only one job. For example, testosterone and estrogen have numerous roles affecting many things throughout your body. Testosterone is responsible for much more than helping men grow beards and develop deep voices, and estrogen does far more than influence female sex characteristics. These hormones affect numerous organs and tissues, regulating and participating in countless biochemical processes. Insulin is no different. It has several functions; helping to lower blood sugar is only one of them.

Insulin: One Actor, Many Roles

Totally separate from its effect on blood sugar, a major role of insulin is in inhibiting lipolysis, the breakdown of fat. (*Lipo* means fat; *lysis* means breaking apart.) Yes, you read that correctly: Insulin makes it much harder to burn fat. Think of insulin as a security guard that stands outside your fat cells to make sure the fat doesn't escape. If you want to lose body fat, it has to be released from storage in your fat cells so it can be sent to other cells that can use it for fuel. You can't burn fat if it won't even come out of your fat cells.

It's difficult to burn fat when you have chronically high insulin. (You'll still burn a *little* fat. The human body isn't binary; its internal processes are never fully on or off. It's more like a seesaw, with certain things happening more often or to a greater extent while others happen less often or to a smaller extent.) Compared to fats and proteins, carbohydrates affect blood sugar the most, so carbohydrates affect insulin the most, too. Think of insulin as putting the brakes on fat-burning and pressing the gas pedal on burning carbs. So, if carbs raise insulin the most, then carbs have the most powerful effect on limiting your body's fat-burning. And if you're not burning fat, it goes into storage.

If you've had a hard time losing weight, it could be that your body is especially sensitive to carbohydrates—meaning that your blood sugar or insulin rises very high after you've consumed carbs (especially refined carbs). Maybe you've spent years following a high-carb diet and trying to keep your fat intake low. But what you didn't know is that those carbs—and their effect on insulin—kept you in carb-burning mode. If you added exercise to the mix, things might have gone like this: eat carbs, burn carbs, refuel and replenish with carbs. When did fat ever enter the picture? It didn't! No wonder this strategy fails so often. It sounds great in theory, but it's a disaster in practice.

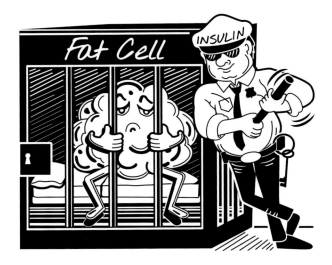

Fig 3.1: Insulin is like a security guard that stands outside your fat cells and makes sure the fat doesn't escape. No wonder it can be so difficult to lose weight on a high-carb diet!

When it comes to fat, insulin is a storage hormone. It promotes storage of excess food energy as fat and then keeps that fat locked away. From this perspective, you can think of insulin as influencing the *growth of* your fat stores. Insulin is a growth promoter in other cells and tissues, too. Chronically elevated insulin is the main driver behind benign prostate hypertrophy (BPH, aka enlarged prostate gland) in men and polycystic ovarian syndrome (PCOS) in women. High insulin makes cysts grow in the ovaries. It also results in skin tags—excessive growth of skin.

Insulin and Hypertension

High insulin levels are also a major factor in hypertension (high blood pressure) and gout—conditions you might be living with even if you don't have diabetes and aren't overweight. Remember, insulin does much more than lower your blood sugar. One of the other things it does is signal your kidneys to hold on to sodium. In the process of filtering your blood, healthy kidneys hang on to just the right amount of sodium and remove the excess to be excreted in your urine. When your insulin is high, though, your kidneys retain more sodium, and in the human body, water follows sodium. More sodium retention means more water retention. More water retention means bloating, edema, swollen legs and ankles, and especially higher blood pressure. (Your blood is mostly water. When your kidneys keep more sodium in your blood because insulin directs them to, there's more water in your blood, making your blood volume larger. A larger volume of blood flowing through the same area of blood vessels means higher pressure.)

Consequently, people with hypertension are counseled to follow a low-sodium diet. The problem with this advice, though, is that sodium is an essential nutrient, despite the bad reputation it's gotten over the past few decades. You would die without it. The truth is that diets that are too *low* in sodium may be more dangerous than diets that are high in sodium. So why would you want to skimp on something so important? Instead of taking in less sodium, focus on why your body is holding on to too much of it and correct *that* problem.

Some of the most commonly prescribed medications for hypertension are diuretics. These types of drugs help your body get rid of excess water. Unfortunately, they don't treat the problem; they only deal with the symptom. They address the effect while ignoring the cause. If the cause is your body holding on to too much sodium and water, and the cause of *that* is high insulin, then the logical and most effective thing to do is to bring your insulin level down.

Stress is another factor in high blood pressure, partly because of how chronic stress affects the nervous system. There are different aspects of your nervous system. The part called the *sympathetic nervous system* is responsible for the "fight-or-flight" feelings you experience when you're in an immediately stressful situation, such as when you're stuck in an aggravating traffic jam, having a heated argument with your spouse, or racing against a tight deadline at work. Under these circumstances, your body floods itself with glucose because your brain is sending messages that there's some kind of acute emergency, and you need that quick burst of energy to stay and fight or run for your life. The result is that even when you're not eating much carbohydrate, stress can keep your blood sugar higher than it would be in the absence of stress.

This surge of glucose in the blood isn't a bad thing. In fact, in a life-or-death situation, it's good; it literally keeps you alive. The problem is, people rarely face immediately life-threatening situations in the twenty-first century, but the human brain is evolutionarily hardwired to *interpret* certain circumstances as dangerous—like those deadlines and traffic jams. Some people are as cool as cucumbers regardless of what's going on around them, but others are especially sensitive to stress and live in a constant state of high alert, which can cause blood sugar and insulin to be higher.

Elevated insulin affects the sympathetic nervous system, even in the absence of stress. Insulin affects numerous other hormones and physical structures in the body, including the blood vessels. High insulin causes blood vessels to tighten and constrict, and constricted blood vessels mean higher blood pressure.

Insulin and Gout

The story is similar for gout. Gout flares happen when a compound called *uric acid* builds up in the joints and forms solid crystals. If you or someone you know suffers from gout, then you know it's very painful. Typically, healthy kidneys hold on to the right amount of uric acid and filter out the rest—much like they hang on to the right amount of sodium—but high insulin levels cause your kidneys to hold on to more uric acid than normal.

The parallels between sodium, uric acid, kidney function, and your overall health don't end there. Uric acid comes from the breakdown of something called *purines*. Purines are nitrogen-containing compounds that your body produces, and they are also found in foods—protein-rich foods, in particular. Certain proteins—such as shellfish, red meat, and organ meats (liver, kidney)—are higher in purines than others, which is why people who suffer from gout are advised to avoid these foods. However, red meat and shellfish are among the most nutrient-dense foods in the modern diet. Aside from being great sources of complete protein, they're loaded with B vitamins, iron, zinc, selenium, and other critical vitamins and minerals. You can get these nutrients from other foods, but red meat and seafood provide them in exceptionally high amounts and in forms your body can absorb more easily than others, and you don't need to avoid them if you have gout.

If gout flares come from an accumulation of uric acid crystals in your joints, and elevated insulin causes your kidneys to hang on to too much uric acid, then rather than avoiding foods whose breakdown creates uric acid, you might be better served by keeping your insulin level lower. Plus, uric acid doesn't exist to trigger gout attacks and cause you pain. It's an antioxidant, so you wouldn't want to be entirely without uric acid in your body. Too much is a problem, but you do need some. And "too much" uric acid comes from too much insulin. The truth is, if you have gout, you can enjoy *more* red meat and seafood—as long as you keep your *carbohydrate* intake low.

Insulin and Sexual Function

What else does insulin affect? I mentioned erectile dysfunction earlier and explained the connection to chronically high blood sugar. Even when blood sugar is normal, high insulin can put a damper on men's sexual function and overall health. Insulin affects testosterone, and not in a good way. Chronically high insulin is one of the culprits behind the epidemic of "low T" that affects so many men. High levels of insulin cause men's bodies to convert some of their testosterone to estrogen, with all the effects you might expect, including the development and enlargement of breast tissue. Enlarged breasts in men aren't inherently harmful, although some people find them aesthetically unpleasing. The real problem is what breast enlargement in men indicates is going on internally: chronically high insulin and abnormally elevated estrogen. Some of the supplements and pharmaceutical drugs designed to raise testosterone levels do so by reducing the conversion of testosterone to estrogen. However, you could do this naturally—and for free—by keeping your insulin level low and losing body fat.

I explained earlier that insulin has a big role in making it easier to gain body fat and harder to lose it. To add insult to injury with regard to men's health, fat tissue secretes estrogen, so while elevated insulin puts up a roadblock to fat loss, it rolls out the red carpet for increased estrogen coming from growing fat stores. To be clear, men normally produce some estrogen; it's not solely a female hormone. But women produce much more estrogen than men do, and things go awry when men produce a lot more of it than is biologically normal.

Oddly enough, however, high insulin has the opposite effect in women: Chronically elevated insulin in women leads to *more* testosterone. Nowhere is this demonstrated more clearly than in women who suffer from PCOS. Many of the signs and symptoms of PCOS result from the direct influence of insulin on other hormones. Most women with PCOS have elevated testosterone, which leads to the acne, oily skin, and facial and body hair that often come along for the ride. (Women produce testosterone, but much less than men do, and this hormone train goes off track when women produce too much insulin.)

Insulin also affects the hormones that regulate the menstrual cycle, resulting in irregular periods and irregular or absent ovulation. PCOS is the most common cause of infertility in women in the industrialized world, and it's almost entirely due to chronically high insulin. The good news here is that it's also almost entirely fixable: bring insulin levels down and keep them low. Part 2 explains how to do that.

By the way, did you know you don't even have to have cysts in your ovaries to be diagnosed with PCOS? That's only one of the signs, and you can be diagnosed with PCOS without them—because even though the name is *polycystic* ovarian syndrome, only some women with the condition have cystic ovaries. In some women, insulin acts as a growth promoter to stimulate the growth of cysts, but in other women, this effect is absent, whereas other effects—such as elevated testosterone, facial hair, and lack of ovulation—are present.

Metabolic Syndrome: Insulin Run Amok

You've probably heard the phrases *insulin resistance* and *metabolic syndrome*. Maybe you've been diagnosed with one of them. They're basically the same thing. In fact, metabolic syndrome used to be called *insulin resistance syndrome*.
I wish it still had that name because chronically high insulin is the cause of metabolic syndrome. Calling it *insulin resistance* syndrome puts the spotlight where it belongs: on insulin.

> " Chronically **high insulin** is the cause of **metabolic syndrome**. Calling it *insulin resistance syndrome* puts the spotlight where it belongs: **on insulin**.

An even more accurate name might be *chronic hyperinsulinemia syndrome. Insulin resistance* is a fuzzy term. Ask ten doctors to give a precise definition, and you'll get ten different answers and ten different recommendations for what to do about it. But call it *chronic hyperinsulinemia*, and its meaning is built right into the phrase:

Chronic: often or all the time
Hyper: high
Insulin: the hormone insulin
–emia: in the blood

Chronic hyperinsulinemia means that the level of insulin in your blood is too high, too often. Now the solution becomes self-evident: lower your insulin level. You can do this in different ways; the most effective method is to cut way back on the amount of carbohydrate you eat.

However, because *metabolic syndrome* is the commonly accepted term right now, I'm using that. Metabolic syndrome is diagnosed by assessing the following criteria. If three or more of these conditions apply to you or you are taking medication for them, you can technically be diagnosed with metabolic syndrome:

- Large waist circumference:
    - \> 35 inches (89 centimeters) for women
    - \> 40 inches (102 centimeters) for men

- High triglycerides: > 150 mg/dL (1.7 mmol/L)
- Low HDL:
    - < 50 mg/dL (1.3 mmol/L) for women
    - < 40 mg/dL (1.04 mmol/L) for men

- Hypertension: ≥ 130/85 mmHg
- Elevated fasting glucose: ≥ 100 mg/dL (5.6 mmol/L)

Take a good look at those five criteria. Something you might expect to be on the list is missing: weight. That's right; body weight is not part of the diagnostic criteria for metabolic syndrome because you can have this cluster of signs and symptoms at any weight. Let me say that again because it's important: *You can have metabolic syndrome even if you are not overweight.* (Conversely, being overweight does not automatically imply that you do have metabolic syndrome.) You might have noticed something else missing—something surprising: insulin. The diagnostic criteria for a condition driven by chronically high insulin do not even include a measurement of insulin! As odd as this seems, there may be a reason for it—one I'll get to soon.

It's Not About Weight

I've talked a lot about diabetes because I'm an internal medicine physician, but I'm also an obesity medicine specialist, and these are the top two reasons people come to my clinic: to treat type 2 diabetes and to lose weight.

Here's the thing: Metabolic syndrome isn't exclusive to people who are carrying extra weight or who have obesity. Type 2 diabetes and obesity go hand-in-hand so often that there's a new word to describe the two of them together: *diabesity*. But both type 2 diabetes and metabolic syndrome can and do occur in people all across the body weight spectrum. Not everyone with obesity has type 2 diabetes or metabolic syndrome, and not everyone with type 2 diabetes or metabolic syndrome is overweight.

What does this mean in the real world? It means that being at a normal weight and even having normal blood sugar levels doesn't mean someone is metabolically healthy. Gaining excessive body fat is more of a *symptom* of metabolic problems than it is a cause. Many people with the underlying problem of chronic hyperinsulinemia pack on the pounds, but some don't. Some men develop BPH (enlarged prostate); others don't. Some women develop PCOS; others don't. Some people will have hypertension; others won't. The same root cause—chronically high insulin—leads to different problems in different people. But if these problems all have the same cause, then they all have the same solution: bring insulin levels down.

> " There are different ways to lower insulin, **but the most effective** is to cut way back on the amount of **carbohydrate** you **eat**.

Even if you don't have excess weight to lose, cutting carbs is important if you're living with any of the many issues caused by chronically elevated insulin. Controlling blood sugar is a huge part of staying healthy over the long term, and doctors and nutritionists are right to educate their patients and clients about this. But there's a gap between the focus on blood sugar and recognizing the importance of insulin. Millions of people have normal blood sugar but chronically high insulin, and they and their doctors may have a false sense of security about their metabolic health.

For people who do have high blood sugar (people with type 2 diabetes or prediabetes), some of the medications used to help control blood sugar can make the insulin problem worse. It sounds counterintuitive, but many people with type 2 diabetes and prediabetes don't have too little insulin; they have too much. If their blood sugar is high, you would think the reason is that they're not producing enough insulin. Many of them have plenty of insulin, however, and the problem is that their bodies are not responding to it properly. (This is one of those ten different definitions you might get for "insulin resistance.") Giving them insulin injections helps to lower their blood sugar at the moment, but it doesn't do anything to address why their bodies aren't effectively using the more-than-adequate insulin they're already producing. Beyond insulin injections, other types of diabetes drugs stimulate the body to make even more of its own insulin. Either way, the result is putting additional insulin into a system that already has more than enough.

And remember that apart from its effect on blood sugar, insulin is a storage hormone. It puts fat into fat cells and helps it stay there, which is why many people with type 2 diabetes who use insulin injections to control their blood sugar gain weight and find it difficult to lose any.

You can see now that type 2 diabetes and obesity are only two of the many issues that come from chronic hyperinsulinemia. This highlights a flaw in how metabolic health and carbohydrate sensitivity are typically assessed. The diagnostic criteria for type 2 diabetes are based on one thing only: blood glucose. It can be diagnosed by a fasting blood glucose test, hemoglobin A1c, or the response to an oral glucose tolerance test, which involves drinking pure liquid glucose and having your blood sugar measured at intervals up to two hours afterward. Insulin levels are not factored in at all, but remember, metabolic syndrome and all the negative effects on health that result from chronic hyperinsulinemia are caused by just that: the high insulin, whether or not your blood glucose is high. (High blood glucose and high insulin together make things even worse, but all by itself, high insulin in the absence of high glucose is the driver of many major health issues.)

How do you know if you have high insulin? You can have your fasting insulin level tested just like you can with glucose. However, as is the case for fasting glucose, testing fasting insulin has shortcomings. What's true for glucose is also true for insulin: many people have a normal fasting level, but after they eat a meal—especially if it's a high-carb meal—insulin rises abnormally high and stays high for hours.

More advanced ways to assess insulin levels in response to eating carbohydrate exist, but there are plenty of clues that you likely have chronically high insulin even without these specialized tests. If you're living with any of the conditions known to be caused or exacerbated by high insulin, there's a high probability you have elevated insulin and are exquisitely sensitive to carbohydrates. If you meet three or more of the criteria for metabolic syndrome, it's a safe bet you have chronic hyperinsulinemia, and some doctors now believe meeting only two of them is enough to indicate high insulin. You can also bank on carbohydrate sensitivity or chronically elevated insulin if you're living with PCOS, nonalcoholic fatty liver disease, hypoglycemia, gout, skin tags, BPH, unexplained hypertension, or erectile dysfunction, or if you've struggled to lose weight despite exercising and following a low-fat (*high-carb*) diet.

> You can **bank** on **carbohydrate sensitivity** or **chronically elevated insulin** if you're living with PCOS, nonalcoholic fatty liver disease, hypoglycemia, gout, skin tags, BPH, unexplained hypertension, or erectile dysfunction, or if you've **struggled to lose weight despite exercising** and following a **low-fat diet**.

No Carbs, No Way?

Don't panic!

If chronically high blood sugar or insulin causes so many problems and cutting way back on dietary carbohydrates is effective for keeping blood sugar and insulin levels lower, does everyone need to follow a strict low-carb diet? No. Many people do follow this type of diet, and it's a good way to stay healthy over the long term, but it's not the only way. Carbohydrate tolerance varies a lot among different people. Just like there are very tall people, very short people, and people at all different heights in between, some people will do best by keeping their total carb intake very low, whereas others can be a little more liberal. But no one—*no one*—needs to eat sugar.

From Obesity, PCOS, and Infertility to Motherhood and a Healthy Weight

"Miraculous things started happening on keto."

I've been asked to share my story a number of times. I've always been rather resistant to it because it's MY journey. A journey that has not been linear, so I don't really feel like I'm even close to an expert on it. I have had lots of successes and just as many failures, if not more.

My story pretty much begins at birth. I have battled my weight all of my life, and my weight, size, and body image is something I've never stopped thinking about. Every year when I blew out my birthday candles, "to not be fat" was always my wish.

My story also includes multiple enrollments in a popular commercial weight-loss program based on counting calories and points—the first time when I was eight years old. This program did not work for me any of the times I tried, even though I followed the prescribed plan.

I always knew something wasn't quite right with me, but I was finally diagnosed with PCOS at the age of twenty-four. I was dealing with some pretty severe symptoms, and it was at this time that I hit my all-time highest weight. I was also in the highest number that most clothing stores carried in the plus-sized section. I was uncomfortable on airplanes and in movie theaters, amusement parks, and even my bathtub.

Fortunately, with the PCOS diagnosis came some answers. I read two books about low-carb diets and learned that this way of eating could alleviate PCOS symptoms.

Fast-forward seven months: I'd lost 70 pounds (32 kg), and my fertility had returned. I managed to conceive our second child, which was incredible considering the PCOS diagnosis just a couple of years prior. With another pregnancy came a lot of weight gain. Low-carb eating took a backseat when I was pregnant and nursing. The weight came back. Not all of it, but most of it.

If you're thinking there's no way you're ever giving up certain sweet or starchy foods, stay with me. You might not have to. Remember the GPS I talked about earlier in the book? The route that's best for you depends on where you're starting from and where you'd like to go. The more excess weight you're carrying or the more out of control your diabetes, blood pressure, joint pain, fatigue, or other health issues, the more strictly you'll have to stick to your route. On the other hand, if you're pretty close to where you want to be, then you have the flexibility to take a few detours, and if you're already there, you have more freedom to explore the terrain and enjoy the scenery. If you don't know where you're starting from, Chapter 6 will help you find the right place to begin.

Each time I've adopted a low-carb lifestyle, I've successfully taken weight off. Unfortunately, I'm like a lot of people who went into it thinking that once the weight was off, I could start eating "normally" again. Now I know that it doesn't work that way.

I should mention that no healthcare professional had ever been remotely helpful in my battle with my weight. Any health issue I may have had over the years was always blamed on my weight, and my weight was always blamed on a poor diet or lack of activity (neither of which I had—except for following the food pyramid, which we now know isn't good).

Three years ago, I'd finally had enough. I started eating low-carb again and eventually learned about the keto diet. It was fairly easy to follow keto, as I'd had so much experience with low-carb. Miraculous things started happening on keto, including hitting my goal weight—the lowest weight of my adult life. I'd lost a total of 155 pounds (70 kg) and maintained that for the better part of a year.

I'm not going to lie. My journey is far from done. I've had some hiccups (in the form of perimenopause) that I'm currently working through. But aside from that, I am in the best health of my life. My biomarkers of health look great. I may not be maintaining my absolute lowest weight at this point, but I'm still in a much better place than I have been for most of my life.

I will keep on keeping on. I'm firmly and happily entrenched in the world of keto. I weigh, measure, and track my food. I read books, watch videos, listen to podcasts, and attend conferences. Keto/low-carb is what I will do forever. My mindset has changed. It's not a diet, but a lifestyle. Knowing that makes a huge difference.

—Rachel G., Shakopee, MN

CHAPTER 4

A CRASH COURSE IN CARBS

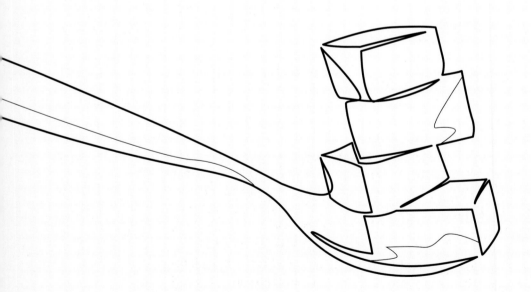

Let's get one thing out of the way right here: Nobody's health ever got worse when they stopped eating sugar. Serious diseases result from severe deficiencies in individual vitamins, minerals, and essential fats or from inadequate protein intake, but there are no diseases caused by a sugar deficiency. *None.*

It's almost impossible to get doctors and dietitians from the different warring nutritional factions to agree on anything. If there's one exception, it's sugar. No matter which diet they're partial to—vegetarian, keto, Mediterranean, vegan, Paleo, low-fat, pescatarian, or some other approach—I can't think of any medical or nutrition professional who would advise a patient to eat more sugar. They do run into trouble, however, when they forget that many seemingly wholesome foods are made from sugar even if they don't look like the white cubes or crystals that likely come to mind when you hear the word *sugar*.

Which brings us to carbohydrates. Remember that carbohydrates have a much bigger effect on your blood sugar and insulin than protein and fat do, so if you're living with an issue related to high blood sugar or insulin, reducing your carbohydrate intake is the most powerful step you can take to start righting your health ship.

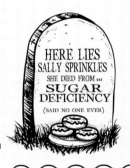

Fig 4.1: No one has ever died from a sugar deficiency.

Aren't There Some Healthy Carbs?

I've already talked about sugar and how it hijacks your appetite, robs your body of nutrients, and wreaks havoc all over your body. But what about other carbohydrates? What about fruit, potatoes, bread, rice, beans, and other sweet and starchy foods? Healthy people all over the world consume these and have for thousands of years. These foods do provide important nutrients, and it would be silly for me to claim that they are the cause of metabolic diseases that only began to get out of control during the last 50 years or so. Carbohydrates are not inherently evil. However, if you're living with a health condition rooted in high blood sugar or insulin, your body doesn't tolerate carbs the way someone's without that condition does—not even natural, whole-food carbs. Something that might be perfectly fine for someone else to eat may not be metabolically safe for you.

> If you're living with an **issue** related to **high blood sugar** or **insulin**, **reducing** your **carbohydrate intake** is the **most powerful step** you can take to start righting your health ship.

There's nothing in high-carbohydrate foods that you can't get from low-carbohydrate foods. For example, you might be used to thinking of orange juice as a good source of vitamin C. And sure, oranges *are* a good source of vitamin C, but you can also get vitamin C from broccoli, tomatoes, and bell peppers—minus the hit to your blood sugar. Bananas are touted as being high in potassium, but you know what's even higher, ounce for ounce? Avocados. And avocados are much lower in carbs and higher in fiber than bananas are. There are no vitamins or minerals that are provided exclusively in high-carb foods—none.

You've heard people say, "You are what you eat," right? Well, that's not quite accurate. You're not what you eat but rather what you *absorb* from what you eat. And when you eat carbohydrates, most of what you absorb is glucose. Table sugar, also called *sucrose*, is half glucose and half fructose. The natural sugar in milk, lactose, is half glucose and half galactose. The carbohydrates in potatoes, beans, and grains—wheat, rice, oats, corn, barley—are almost entirely glucose or sucrose, with small amounts of other carbohydrates. Without adding honey or maple syrup, plain oats don't taste sweet. Because of their bland flavor, no one could blame you for thinking they're not sugary, but they're still very high in carbohydrate. Even though your mouth doesn't perceive them as sweet, oats get broken down into glucose molecules, and this is what you absorb. It doesn't matter whether food tastes sweet or not; what matters is what enters your bloodstream. When you eat high-carbohydrate foods, most of what enters your bloodstream is glucose.

But Isn't Fruit Good for You?

Glucose isn't the only form of sugar. As I mentioned, fructose comes along with glucose in fruit, butternut squash, and certain other sweet and starchy foods. Fructose doesn't have the same effect on raising blood sugar that glucose does, but that doesn't mean it's entirely benign. Because of its effects on the liver, fructose can be harmful in large quantities over the long term. It doesn't affect blood sugar right away like glucose does, but overdoing fructose over the long term can negatively impact insulin sensitivity. Over time, a high intake of fructose interferes with your body's ability to respond to insulin. When this happens, one of two things can result: Your blood sugar will be higher because your cells aren't able to respond to insulin as readily as they did in the past, or your body will pump out a lot more insulin to keep your blood sugar from getting higher. Neither of these is something you want! Plus, fructose never travels by itself; it's found in foods that also contain glucose or sucrose, so you'll reduce your fructose intake automatically when you reduce the total amount of carbohydrate you eat.

Fruit smoothies have been anointed—falsely—with a heavenly health halo, as if they were sent down from above and can do no wrong. Apples, grapes, blueberries, kiwis, bananas, cherries, pineapple, mango, papaya—how can these brightly colored natural foods possibly be bad for you? They practically scream nutrition, and you're supposed to "eat a rainbow" of different foods, right? As I've said, these foods do provide vitamins and minerals, and they're not inherently bad for you. I'm not suggesting fruit salad is the culprit behind the diabesity epidemic, but when you are specifically looking to improve a health condition driven by high blood sugar or insulin, it's best to avoid consuming large amounts of fruit—particularly when the fruits have been squeezed into juice or blended into a smoothie and come in a form you don't even need to chew.

Natural sugar is still sugar. Your pancreas doesn't know the difference between glucose in orange juice and glucose in a sugar-sweetened soda. The merits of eating a variety of vibrantly colored foods are debatable, but if it makes you happy to see a colorful plate in front of you, you can accomplish this just fine with foods that are much lower in carbs: eggplant, asparagus, cauliflower, zucchini, yellow squash, red peppers, purple cabbage, mushrooms, radicchio, radishes, tomatoes.

What About Complex Carbs?

Starches are another category of carbohydrate. These are called *complex carbs* because the individual glucose molecules in them are connected into larger molecules that your body has to break apart before they can enter your bloodstream. They may also contain various types of fiber that slow the digestion of the foods that contain them, so the glucose doesn't enter your bloodstream as quickly as it would from a candy bar, for example. But make no mistake: These foods are still predominantly carbohydrate. Wheat, corn, oats, rice, and other grains contain small amounts of protein and minuscule amounts of fat, but their largest component by far is carbohydrate. Complex or not, digested more slowly or not, what enters your bloodstream is glucose.

While I'm on the topic of starches, *whole grains* is a misnomer. Food manufacturers use this phrase to let you know that the entire kernel or seed—the starch component, the bran and fiber, the protein, and everything else contained in an individual grain—is included in the creation of the food product, like a boxed cereal, a granola bar, crackers, a loaf of bread, or a bag of tortilla chips. But think of whole wheat crackers and compare them to the hard winter wheat berries you find in the bulk bins at health food stores. They look nothing alike. The crackers might have been made using the "whole grain," but the wheat berries were pulverized into flour before being transformed into the crackers you see in the box. They're nothing like their original form, and their effect on your blood sugar is more dramatic than if you were to eat a wheatberry salad where the wheatberries are intact and *truly* whole.

> Wheat, corn, oats, rice, and other grains contain **small amounts** of **protein** and **minuscule amounts** of **fat**, but their largest component by far is **carbohydrate**. Complex or not, digested more slowly or not, what enters your bloodstream is **glucose**.

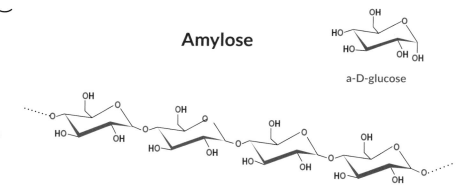

Amylose

a-D-glucose

Fig 4.2: Amylose is one type of starch. All forms of starch and other complex carbohydrates are made up of long strands of glucose molecules and other simple sugars linked together. Your body breaks up these strings during digestion, and the glucose and other sugars are released into your bloodstream.

Image credit: derived from iStock.com/Bacsica

Should I Avoid Processed Foods?

Most healthy ways of eating—whether they're low-carb or not—encourage people to avoid processed foods. There's no formally accepted definition for this phrase in the scientific community, but when people say "processed foods," they're typically referring to packaged food items with long ingredient lists full of words you'd have trouble pronouncing. You can also think of processed foods as something you wouldn't be able to make from scratch in your kitchen.

However, "processing" foods is not automatically a bad thing. It's okay to eat foods that look very different from how they occur naturally. (Salami and prosciutto don't look anything like a live pig, and hamburger patties don't look like cows.) The degree of processing isn't what determines whether certain foods might be problematic for you; the issue is the effect these foods have on your blood sugar and insulin, not to mention your appetite and self-control. If you eat corn on the cob, you'd probably feel satisfied after one or two ears, but if you transform that corn—including using the whole grain—into chips, you might be able to polish off a large bag by yourself, taking in a lot more total calories and carbs. Think again about oats, too. If you had a bowl of steel-cut oatmeal, you'd likely stop after one bowl, but when those same oat groats have been transformed into cereal puffs coated in sugar, you can say goodbye to half the box, right? Toss in some marshmallows or dried blueberries and maybe say goodbye to the whole box.

Trying to distinguish between simple sugars, refined carbs, complex carbs, whole grains, and foods with a lot of added fiber is a losing proposition. Don't get mixed up in this. It's far easier and more effective simply to reduce your intake of carbohydrates across the board. You wouldn't press your luck driving a long distance with your car's gas light on or with the engine overheating in redline territory. Don't tempt fate with your health, either.

Don't be discouraged if you're living with one or more of the conditions you now know are being driven by high blood sugar or insulin. You might have spent many years eating foods that you knew all along weren't great choices for you, or perhaps you consumed lots of whole grains and fruit because you thought you were doing the right thing. You may even have been following orders from a doctor or nutritionist when you were doing this. Whatever brought you to where you are right now, there's good news: food was the problem, but food is also the solution—just not in the way you might think.

> If you've already been **eating less and moving more,** and you've been choosing **whole grain foods** that are **low in fat** and **high in complex carbs** and **natural sugars,** but you're **not getting the results** you want—in fact, you're getting worse— then **stop doing that**. It's time for a **different approach**.

The foods that caused the problem are not the foods that will solve it. It's kind of like this old joke:

Patient: Doctor, it hurts when I do this.

Doctor: *So stop doing that!*

If you've already been "eating less and moving more," and you've been choosing foods that are low in fat and high in complex carbs and natural sugars, but you're not getting the results you want—in fact, you're getting worse—then stop doing that. It's time for a different approach.

From Psoriatic Arthritis, Carb Addiction, and Prediabetes to Food Freedom and a 100-Pound Weight Loss

"It's a celebration of freedom."

My life before keto: *In a word, it SUCKED. I fought weight my whole life, and I was a classic yo-yo dieter. I even battled anorexia as a 16-year-old. I did a commercial weight-loss program twice as well. I went on every diet in the world, it seemed. I would lose weight only to gain it back, plus I'd pack on 20 additional pounds every time. By the time I had ballooned to 260 pounds (118 kg), I just didn't care anymore. I thought, "I'm just a fat girl, and that's all I'll ever be. Forget it; I'll eat what I want."*

I was very sick with psoriatic arthritis. There were days I couldn't walk from my bed to the bathroom by myself due to the excruciating pain. I once had a flare that affected almost every joint in my body, from my jaws to my toes. This just added to my depression and apathy. I had nothing left to fight with. I was on several drugs, including methotrexate (a form of chemotherapy), and I was also taking oxycodone like candy, just to be able to function. I was on mega doses of prednisone as well, which may have contributed to my prediabetes. It wasn't until I had the prediabetes diagnosis and was in such pain from my knees that I knew I had to do something drastic. I didn't want to be diabetic, and I needed surgery to help my knee pain. I was so heavy that no orthopedic surgeon would operate until I lost weight. I didn't know how in the world I was going to correct my issues.

Being a person of faith, I did the only thing I knew to do when you're at your wits' end: I got down on my knees and prayed for God to help me. I still didn't know how I was going to approach my weight loss at that point. The next day I was scrolling through Instagram, and an ad for Audible came up. The book advertised was about how the hormone insulin was the key to controlling weight. Being that I was prediabetic, the mention of insulin immediately got my attention. I downloaded the book immediately and devoured it. The whole time I listened, I kept saying to myself, "This is ME! This is ME!" So after that, I began to research everything I could find about keto. I'm a researcher by nature, so I pretty much became obsessed with any information I could get on the subject. After reading the book about insulin and obesity, I found some keto-oriented doctors online, and that's when my life was forever changed. I took the plunge into the keto world. I had keto flu symptoms for about four days, but it wasn't as bad as some people make it sound. I was over it pretty quickly.

My life now: *It's fantastic. I'm off all prescription meds—all of them. I'm in the best physical shape of my life, and I have freedom from the addiction to carbs. It's true freedom not to be a slave to those controlling foods anymore. I don't think about food very much at all. I don't get hungry. I do intermittent fasting most every day. As I went along my journey, I gave up other things that I knew were not good for me. Caffeine and* *artificial sweeteners, to name a couple. I won't say I never have them, but it's a very rare occasion. As of January 10, 2020, I had maintained a weight loss of more than 100 pounds (45 kg) for a year. I've never maintained any weight loss ever. I am victorious in my battle with my weight and my health. (Yes, anyone who's lost that much weight remembers the exact date they started keto!)*

Medical doctors: *Not helpful for me! I went to a new primary care doctor because the one I had seen previously had moved. I was having trouble with hair loss, fatigue, and coldness. I have Hashimoto's thyroid disease but had not experienced a flare in years, probably because I was on a biologic medicine, and when I came off of it, the Hashimoto's flared up. I knew what was wrong with me. I've had it for 20 years. I asked her to do a full thyroid panel, but she refused and only tested TSH and T4, plus a cholesterol panel. I told her that I had lost about 85 pounds (38 kg). She asked me how, and I said keto and intermittent fasting. You would have thought I said I was drinking gasoline or something! She said the reason my hair was falling out was that I was not eating a balanced diet. I told her I was eating more vegetables than I had ever eaten in my life, and I was eating no processed food of any kind. This did not satisfy her. When my cholesterol panel came back, she immediately wanted to put me on a statin and told me point-blank that if I didn't stop eating keto, I was going to die. I fired her after that and didn't go back. After going to a different doctor, who performed a full thyroid testing panel, I found out that my hypothyroidism was indeed raging, which was responsible for most of the symptoms I'd been having. Once I was on thyroid hormone, I was no longer cold all the time, the fatigue is no longer an issue, and my hair stopped falling out. Imagine that!*

Straying from keto: *I aim to stay in ketosis all the time. Only on rare occasions do I not. I enjoy wine from time to time, and even if something I eat or drink puts me out of ketosis, I typically get right back in because my body is fat-adapted now. I have not eaten a piece of bread, a slice of pizza, any pasta, potatoes, or starchy vegetables in almost 2 years. I just don't go there. It's an addiction, and it only takes once. I'm NOT going back down that path. I'm free, and I'm going to stay that way. I eat only real whole foods. I don't feel the need for all those bad carbs anymore, and I don't crave them. I truly don't. I do sometimes crave sweets, and there are keto-friendly alternatives for that. One of the main reasons I started my keto group was for accountability. How can I lead the group if I'm constantly falling off the wagon? So, I don't go there. I stay committed to keto to be strong for the others who are not yet free and to keep myself in check. Motivating others keeps me motivated. My "ketoversary" was on January 2, 2020. It's been more than two years now. It was a celebration of freedom.*

—Kim C., Braselton, GA

PART 2

THE ADAPT YOUR LIFE DIET

CHAPTER 5

INTRO TO CARBOHYDRATE CONTROL

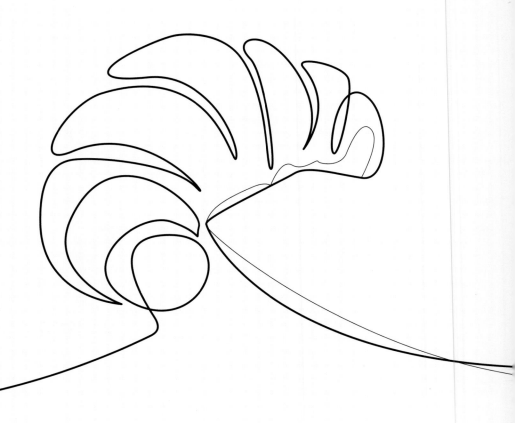

Let's get back to our road trip. When you're on the road, you care only about your destination. There are thousands of other drivers on the highway with you, but you don't need to know where they're headed; you only need to think about *your* route, *your* next turn. Those thousands of other drivers didn't start where you started, and they're probably not headed where you're headed, so *their* routes are irrelevant to you. It doesn't matter how many miles they've already covered or how close they are to their destinations because they're on their journeys, and you're on yours. Besides, they're driving different cars and probably listening to different music. For example, maybe some of them are driving brand-new sports cars that hum along and make them feel like they're coasting on clouds, whereas your car might have a lot more miles on it and need new tires and shocks. Maybe you need to be more careful to steer clear of potholes. The point is, keep your eyes on the road ahead of you, and don't compare your trip to anyone else's.

> If you're living with a **health condition** rooted in **high blood sugar** or **insulin**, your body **doesn't tolerate carbs** the way another person's body does if they don't have that condition. Something that might be **perfectly fine for someone else** to eat may not be **metabolically safe** for **you**.

Begin with the End in Mind

Where you start and how far you are from your destination will help determine the best route for you to take. If you can't imagine summer without the juice of a ripe peach running down your chin, maybe you don't have to. And if you can't imagine a leisurely Sunday breakfast without hash browns or home fries alongside your bacon and eggs, maybe you don't have to do that. Similarly, if you have a lot of weight to lose and you've assumed you'll have to give up juicy steaks, fatty pork chops, and your favorite cheeses in favor of bland rice cakes and salad with no dressing, maybe you don't have to do that, either.

There are millions (billions, actually) of healthy people all around the world who are lean, active, and living well who do not follow low-carb diets. Very low-carb approaches are not necessarily required to be in your best health. If you're already healthy and simply want to stay that way, your carbohydrate threshold—the amount of carbohydrate your body can handle and allow you to remain in good health—is higher than that of someone who's sick or very overweight and wants to reclaim their health. The strategy and tactics needed to fix a problem after it already exists are not the same approach that might prevent the problem from happening in the first place. Different situations call for different approaches. (You'll learn more about this in Chapters 7 through 9, which cover the three phases of the ADAPT Your Life Diet.)

It's not that low-fat diets don't work, or that any approach other than reducing your carb intake can't be effective for you. Out on that road trip, you'll see Fords, Toyotas, Subarus, Chevrolets, Jeeps, Porsches, Ferraris, BMWs, Teslas, and other brands of cars. They all work. They can all get someone from point A to point B, but they come with different features. Certain brands are better suited for certain kinds of driving experiences. If you're carrying a lot of excess weight or you're dealing with a metabolic condition driven by high blood sugar or insulin, keeping carbs low will give you the most efficient (and probably the quickest and easiest) path to better health. On the other hand, if you're already healthy and want to stay that way, you don't have to keep carbs quite as low as someone who's trying to recover their health. Different kind of driving experience, different kind of car. Different health situation, different approach to diet.

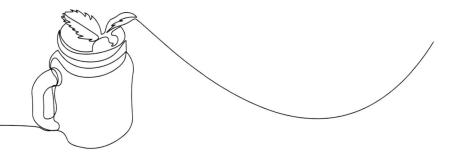

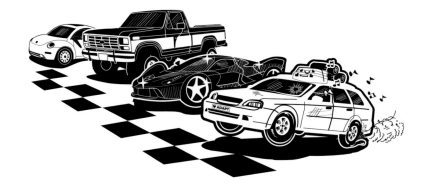

Fig 5.1: Different driving experience, different car. Different health situation, different diet.

What About a Low-Glycemic Diet?

As I'll discuss in the next few chapters, the ADAPT Your Life Diet is about customizing the total amount of carbohydrate you eat. If you're wondering whether you could follow a low-glycemic diet and get the same results as you will with the ADAPT Your Life Diet, your mind is in the right place. You're thinking about the relevant issue, which is controlling blood sugar. However, low-glycemic diets are a mixed bag.

The glycemic index is a rough estimate of how quickly a particular food or beverage will raise your blood sugar. The glycemic index (GI) is determined based on giving people a serving of food that provides 50 grams of carbohydrate and measuring their blood sugar over the next two hours. (The number is compared to the response to pure glucose, which has a glycemic index of 100. The higher the number is—the closer it is to pure glucose—the more quickly it raises your blood sugar.) This is misleading for several reasons. First, there's a lot of individual variation in how different foods and beverages affect people's blood sugar. One person's high-fiber whole-grain cereal is another's white bread with grape jelly. In other words, what's metabolically safe for another person to consume might not be a good idea for you, especially if you're already living with a condition related to high blood sugar. Just because a food or beverage has a low glycemic index doesn't mean it's low glycemic for *you*.

The second problem with the glycemic index is that it's unrealistic when it comes to portion sizes. Because it's based on the blood sugar response to a serving of food that provides 50 grams of carbohydrate, depending on how carbohydrate-dense the food is, the serving size used to determine the GI in test subjects could have been either abnormally large or small. For example, watermelon has a relatively high GI of 76, but because it's mostly water with a little bit of fiber, you would have to consume an incredibly large amount of watermelon to get 50 grams of carbohydrate. The GI of apple juice is about half of that—only 41, but 1 cup (237 ml) of apple juice provides 28 grams of carbohydrate, and many people would get a refill—maybe two refills—giving them more than 50 grams of carbohydrate before they've finished the second cup.

> " There's a **lot** of **individual variation** in how different foods and beverages affect people's **blood sugar**. One person's **high-fiber**, whole-grain cereal is another's **white bread with grape jelly**. Just because a food has a **low** glycemic index **doesn't mean** it's low glycemic for **you**.

Glycemic *load* (GL) is a slightly more helpful concept, but it's still too flawed to use as a guide for your health. Unlike the GI, the GL takes typical portion sizes into account, which makes the impact on blood sugar more realistic, but it still isn't solid enough for you to rely on. What is a "typical" portion? Some of the online GL charts list the GL of jelly beans based on a 1-ounce serving (28 grams). One ounce of *jelly beans*! Right! When was the last time anyone stopped after 1 *ounce* of candy? A serving of maple syrup is listed as 1 tablespoon. Don't make me laugh!

> " The **easiest** way to **control** the **glycemic impact** of your entire diet is to **consume** foods and **beverages** that are **low** in total **carbohydrate**, and only those foods and beverages. When your diet consists solely of foods and beverages that are **low in carbs** to begin with, you **don't** have to **worry** about the **glycemic impact**.

Those arguments are already strong enough to support not trying to follow a low-glycemic diet, but if you need another reason, be aware that the glycemic index is based on eating one food by itself. For example, eating a potato without butter, sour cream, or an accompanying steak. Eating cereal without milk, or spaghetti without sauce and meatballs. The problem here is that combining foods changes your glycemic response to them, so, right off the bat, glycemic measurements aren't all that realistic because they don't take into account how people eat meals in the real world.

Since different foods affect people differently, the glycemic index and glycemic load can be misleading. If you want to get really technical, you could get a handheld meter for measuring blood sugar (called a *glucometer*) to test the effects of individual foods. However, you'd have to test them over and over in all the different combinations you would normally eat them. For example, bread with butter, bread as a sandwich with turkey and mayo inside, and bread cut up and baked as croutons for a salad. You'd drive yourself nuts trying to ferret out every possible factor affecting how *your body* responds to individual foods.

If you need one more reason to ditch a low-glycemic approach, I'll give it to you, and this one may be the most important. Keep in mind that neither glycemic index nor load takes insulin into account. Remember, you can have normal blood sugar after consuming a certain food or beverage, but sometimes this normal blood sugar happens at the expense of high insulin. Flooding your body with insulin to maintain normal blood sugar is not a trade-off you want to make.

Instead of messing with all this uncertainty, you could keep things dead simple and keep your carbohydrate intake low across the board. The easiest way to control the glycemic impact of your entire diet is to consume foods and beverages that are low in total carbohydrate, and *only* those foods and beverages. No confusion, no math, no headaches. When your diet consists solely of foods and beverages that are low in carbohydrate to begin with, you don't have to worry about the glycemic impact.

Think again about the road trip. Would you follow a map that was right only sometimes? A map that sometimes leads you to a bridge that's still being built or a road that's closed for construction? You could drive yourself off a cliff or straight into the ocean. No, thank you! Instead, how about sticking to a route that will get you to your destination every time with the fewest wrong turns and hiccups along the way?

What's worked in my clinic for more than two decades is the simplest and most direct route: keep all carbs low, period. In the next chapter, you'll determine how low you should go when getting started based on your health history, current situation, medical circumstances, and goals.

Buckle up; it's time for you to get in the driver's seat.

CHAPTER 6

FINDING YOUR CARB THRESHOLD

The ADAPT Your Life Diet is based around the *total amount of carbohydrate* you will be eating each day. If you're looking to lose a large amount of weight or you're currently living with certain medical conditions, the lower your total carbohydrate intake will need to be for you to reach your goals quickly and efficiently. If you're already satisfied with your weight and you're in good health, the more generous you can be with carbohydrates.

What Do You Mean by "Total Carbs"?

If you've ever tried a low-carb diet before or even just read about them, you might have come across the term *net carbs*. Net carbs are calculated by taking the total grams of carbohydrate in a food and subtracting the grams of fiber and sugar alcohols. Some low-carb programs allow you to count net carbs to get your carbohydrate allowance for the day. The reason they do this is because your body doesn't absorb fiber, so it doesn't affect blood sugar or insulin the way other forms of carbohydrate do. However, in more than twenty years of clinical practice, I've found that some types of sugar alcohols do affect blood sugar, and, in rare circumstances, even fiber can have an effect for some people—enough of an effect that it's best just to count total carbohydrates.

In case you're unfamiliar with sugar alcohols, let me explain a little about them. Sugar alcohols are compounds that give foods a sweet taste, but because they're not actually sugar, food manufacturers can use them for sweetening products they want to market as "sugar-free" or as having "no added sugar." So, sugar alcohols are used as sweeteners, but they have a smaller impact on blood sugar and insulin than regular sugar does. Note that I said a *smaller* impact rather than *no* impact. There are several different types of sugar alcohols, and they're a distinct category on nutrition facts labels. You can recognize them by their names, which end in –itol: maltitol, mannitol, sorbitol, xylitol, and erythritol. (See the frequently asked questions in Chapter 11 for how to read a food label and find the total carbs.) Some varieties affect glucose and insulin more than others, and not all people have the same tolerance to these compounds.

When you're following the ADAPT Your Life Diet, keep things simple and just count total carbs so you don't have to deal in guesswork and unpredictability.

The Phases of the ADAPT Your Life Diet

The ADAPT Your Life Diet has three phases, each defined by a range of total carbohydrates. Phase 1 includes 20 total grams of carbohydrate per day or fewer. Phase 2 increases this to 50 total grams of carbohydrate per day or fewer, and Phase 3 is the most relaxed at 150 total grams of carbohydrate per day or fewer. I've deliberately said "or fewer" because the total carbohydrate grams for each phase is not a target to aim for, but rather, a limit to stay under. When you're following Phase 1, you may have *up to* 20 total grams of carbohydrate per day. This doesn't mean you *need* to have 20 total grams; it's okay to have *less* than the total amount permitted. You might find that on some days you've consumed only 10 or 15 total grams, and that's fine. You don't need to eat anything extra to get to 20 total grams. The same is true for Phases 2 and 3: In Phase 2, you may have *up to* 50 total grams of carbs per day, but if it's bedtime and you've had just 35 or 40 grams, you don't need to eat more carbohydrate to hit 50. For Phase 3, you may have *up to* 150 total grams of carbs per day, but it's okay to have less than that.

Determining the Right Phase for You

The following table helps point you toward the phase of the ADAPT Your Life Diet—and the total amount of carbohydrate—that's right for you to start with. I'm saying "start with" because you might be able to transition from one phase to another sometime in the future, but when you're just starting, your best results will happen if you stick with the phase you need most.

Mark all the boxes that best describe your current circumstances and then add up the number of marked boxes in each column.

ADAPT Your Life Diet Phases and Daily Total Carbohydrate Limits

	Phase 1 (Up to 20 total grams per day)	Phase 2 (Up to 50 total grams per day)	Phase 3 (Up to 150 total grams per day)
Overweight (BMI 25–29) or obese (BMI ≥ 30)—see the BMI chart to determine your BMI	☐		
Large waist circumference (large abdomen) but not overweight		☐	
Weight regain after bariatric surgery	☐		
Type 2 diabetes or prediabetes	☐		

	Phase 1 (Up to 20 total grams per day)	Phase 2 (Up to 50 total grams per day)	Phase 3 (Up to 150 total grams per day)
Type 1 diabetes with overweight or obesity*	☐		
Type 1 diabetes but not overweight*		☐	
Irritable bowel syndrome (IBS)	☐		
Migraines	☐		
Hypoglycemia	☐		
Brain fog	☐		
Lipedema or lymphedema	☐		
Hypertension (high blood pressure) plus other health issues	☐		
Hypertension with no other health issues		☐	
Gout plus other health issues	☐		
Gout with no other health issues		☐	
Heartburn (aka acid reflux or GERD)	☐		
Nonalcoholic fatty liver disease ("fatty liver")	☐		
Chronic kidney disease	☐		
Chronic fatigue syndrome or low energy all the time	☐		
Fibromyalgia	☐		
Skin tags	☐		
Adult acne, eczema, or psoriasis plus other health issues	☐		
Adult acne, eczema, or psoriasis with no other health issues		☐	
Mood swings	☐		
Women: Severe PMS and/or menstrual cramps	☐		
Women: PCOS (polycystic ovarian syndrome)	☐		
Women: Post-pregnancy weight loss		☐	
Women: Gestational diabetes		☐	
Men: Enlarged prostate (BPH; benign prostate hypertrophy)		☐	
Men: Erectile dysfunction with no known cause		☐	
Healthy but have a family history of type 2 diabetes		☐	
At your ideal weight; no health issues			☐
At your ideal weight after losing weight on a low-carb, ketogenic, or Paleo-style program		☐	
Slightly overweight but otherwise healthy		☐	
Competitive athlete and at your ideal weight			☐
Competitive athlete but overweight		☐	
Total number of boxes checked			

*See the note regarding type 1 diabetes in Appendix A.

To find your BMI, locate where your height and weight intersect; your BMI is listed at the top of that column

BMI	HEALTHY BMI						OVERWEIGHT BMI				
	19	20	21	22	23	24	25	26	27	28	29
4'10"	91	96	100	105	110	115	119	124	129	134	138
4'11"	94	99	104	109	114	119	124	128	133	138	143
5'	97	102	107	112	118	123	128	133	138	143	148
5'1"	100	106	111	116	122	127	132	137	143	148	153
5'2"	104	109	115	120	126	131	136	142	147	153	158
5'3"	107	113	118	124	130	135	141	146	152	158	163
5'4"	110	116	122	128	134	140	145	151	157	163	169
5'5"	114	120	126	132	138	144	150	156	162	168	174
5'6"	118	124	130	136	142	148	155	161	167	173	179
5'7"	121	127	134	140	146	153	159	166	172	178	185
5'8"	125	131	138	144	151	158	164	171	177	184	190
5'9"	128	135	142	149	155	162	169	176	182	189	196
5'10"	132	139	146	153	160	167	174	181	188	195	202
5'11"	136	143	150	157	165	172	179	186	193	200	208
6'	140	147	154	162	169	177	184	191	199	206	213
6'1"	144	151	159	166	174	182	189	197	204	212	219
6'2"	148	155	163	171	179	186	194	202	210	218	225
6'3"	152	160	168	176	184	192	200	208	216	224	232
6'4"	156	164	172	180	189	197	205	213	221	230	238

HEIGHT

WEIGHT (IN POUNDS)

← Reduced Risk   Increased Risk →

Fig 6.1: This chart shows weight in pounds and height in feet and inches. To calculate your BMI using kilograms and meters, use this formula: weight in kilograms divided by height in meters squared (kg/m^2). For example, if you weigh 84 kilograms and your height is 1.57 meters (157 centimeters), your BMI is 84/1.57*1.57 = 34. There are many online calculators that will do the math for you; all you need to do is enter your height and weight.

Image credit: derived from Abhijeet Bhosale/ Shutterstock.com

	OBESITY BMI										EXTREME OBESITY BMI										
30	31	32	33	34	35	36	37	38	39	40	41	42	43	44	45	46	47	48	49	50
143	148	153	158	162	167	172	177	181	186	191	196	201	205	210	215	220	224	229	234	239
148	153	158	163	168	173	178	183	188	193	198	203	208	212	217	222	227	232	237	242	247
153	158	163	169	173	179	184	189	194	199	204	209	215	220	225	230	235	240	245	250	255
158	164	169	174	180	185	190	195	201	206	211	217	222	227	232	238	243	248	254	259	264
164	169	174	180	185	191	196	202	207	213	218	224	229	235	240	246	251	256	262	267	273
169	176	180	186	192	197	203	208	214	220	225	231	237	242	248	254	259	265	270	278	282
174	180	186	192	197	204	209	215	221	227	232	238	244	250	256	262	267	273	279	285	291
180	186	192	198	204	210	216	222	228	234	240	246	252	258	264	270	276	282	288	294	300
186	192	198	204	210	216	223	229	235	241	247	253	260	266	272	278	284	291	297	303	309
191	198	204	211	217	223	230	236	242	249	255	261	268	274	280	287	293	299	306	312	319
197	203	210	216	223	230	236	243	249	256	262	269	276	282	289	295	302	308	315	322	328
203	209	219	223	230	236	243	250	257	263	270	277	284	291	297	304	311	318	324	331	338
209	216	222	229	236	243	250	257	264	271	278	285	292	299	306	313	320	327	334	341	348
215	222	229	236	243	250	257	265	272	279	286	293	301	308	315	322	329	338	343	351	358
221	228	235	243	250	258	265	272	279	287	294	302	309	316	324	331	338	346	353	361	368
227	235	242	250	257	265	272	280	288	295	302	310	318	325	333	340	348	355	363	371	378
233	241	249	256	264	272	280	287	295	303	311	319	326	334	342	350	358	365	373	381	389
240	248	256	264	272	279	287	295	303	311	319	327	335	343	351	359	367	375	383	391	399
246	254	263	271	279	287	295	304	312	320	328	336	344	353	361	369	377	385	394	402	410

WEIGHT (IN POUNDS)

Increased Risk →

Look at your totals in the three columns of the table on pages 60 and 61. The column with the highest number of boxes checked is the ADAPT Your Life Diet phase that's best for you to start with. As you can see, if you're living with numerous health conditions or you're looking to lose a large amount of weight, you'll start with Phase 1. If you're already healthy, active, and fit, and want to maintain this positive status long term, Phase 3 is the place for you. Phase 2 is an in-between stage where many people will find excellent long-term health and well-being.

The phase you start with won't necessarily be where you stay forever. Adjusting your carbohydrate intake is more an art than it is an exact science. Someone who's followed Phase 1 for a while and has resolved their health issues might be able to transition to Phase 2, and someone who starts at Phase 3 might choose to follow Phase 2 for a time if they notice their health or weight trending in a direction they're unhappy with. Someone who starts at Phase 3 can also try Phase 1 if they want to, and a highly motivated person starting at Phase 1 might, over the long term, be able to transition gradually to Phase 3, but they'll most likely experience their best physical and mental health either staying at Phase 1 permanently or transitioning to Phase 2 and staying there. You'll learn the details about all this in the next few chapters.

If your total number in the column for ADAPT Your Life Phase 1 is high, don't feel discouraged! People just like you have had remarkable transformations in each of the conditions listed there—every one of them. Your body is incredibly resilient. When you remove things that harm it and instead give it what it needs to thrive from the ground up—right at the level of your individual cells—you'll be amazed at how well it responds. Some of the issues in the table will improve rapidly when your body receives better nutrition, and your blood sugar and insulin levels are lower. Other issues will take a little longer to respond, but they will respond in time. For things that take a bit longer, be patient, and stay the course. You'll likely experience rapid improvements in other factors, which will keep you motivated to stick with things.

> **Your body** is incredibly **resilient**. When you **remove** things that **harm it** and **instead give it** what it **needs** to thrive from the ground up—right at the level of your individual cells— you'll be amazed at **how well it responds**.

Chapters 7 through 9 will walk you through the details of Phases 1, 2, and 3 of the ADAPT Your Life Diet. If the numbers in your chart point you toward Phase 2 or Phase 3, don't skip reading about Phase 1. It's the foundation that Phases 2 and 3 are built on, so it's important that you understand it. Plus, for reasons I'll explain soon, even if Phase 2 or Phase 3 seems like the right place for you, you may choose to start at Phase 1 to experience unique effects that you might not get at Phase 2 or Phase 3. Everyone *can* follow Phase 1, but not everyone needs to. Even if the chart points you toward Phase 2 or 3, it's not a bad idea to follow Phase 1 for a month or two, so you'll know if there are particular benefits you get from that approach that you don't get after transitioning to one of the other phases. Armed with that knowledge, you can decide if you'd prefer to stay at Phase 2 or 3 or if you feel your best following Phase 1.

Have you ever felt that a doctor or other medical professional was talking *at* you rather than *with* you? Making all the decisions for you so that you had no say in things? The ADAPT Your Life Diet approach is different. All of it is a choice. *Your choice.* You're in the driver's seat here. All I'm doing is helping to navigate. You're the expert regarding your body. Nobody knows you better than you do, and that means you get to decide what you're going to do.

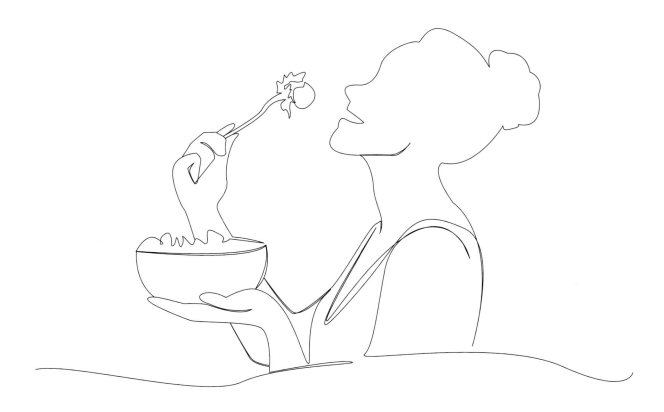

Heart Failure, Fatty Liver, Type 2 Diabetes, Obesity, and IBS to Energetic, Pain-Free, and Full of Life

"My quality of life is at an all-time high. I have never been happier or healthier. To me, this is nothing short of a miracle."

I'll start with the background about my health and weight: I maintained a normal weight and good health for most of my early life—until I had a heart attack at age 39. My left anterior descending artery was more than 90 percent blocked. This particular artery is so infamous for causing sudden death from a heart attack that it's called "the widow maker." A stent was placed in the artery, after which I followed the recommended "cardiac diet" and was also put on antidepressant medication. Over the next few years, while following a low-fat diet and taking lots of meds, I gained a large amount of weight and was diagnosed with a long list of issues, including GERD, irritable bowel syndrome (IBS), nonalcoholic fatty liver disease, and more. The answer was always more meds, and eventually I was diagnosed with prediabetes.

In 2011, I was diagnosed with a form of breast cancer called ductal carcinoma in situ (DCIS) and underwent a bilateral mastectomy. Recovery from this surgery was inhibited by extreme inflammation and fluid accumulation, the severity of which led me to be hospitalized three times. The first time was for an emergency cardiac tamponade caused by pericardial effusion to the tune of an entire liter of fluid. No cause for this was ever identified, and just one month later, I was hospitalized again to remove fluid from one of my lungs.

During this hospital stay, I was diagnosed with mixed connective tissue disease (MCTD), which covers several autoimmune disorders, such as lupus and rheumatoid arthritis. Treatment started with medication, and I saw some small improvements. However, some of the medications I was taking impacted my blood sugar and insulin levels, leading me to full-on type 2 diabetes. In the meantime, my cardiac symptoms progressed: I had shortness of breath, inability to lie down to sleep, edema (fluid retention) in my hands and feet, and extreme fatigue. Most of my doctors pointed to conditions outside their specialty to explain my symptoms: The cardiologist blamed the connective tissue disorder, and the rheumatologist blamed the heart issues. Eventually I ended up in the hospital again after gaining 22 pounds (10 kg) of fluid in three weeks. I was diagnosed with congestive heart failure and sent home after nearly two weeks.

Only a short time later, I collapsed at work, experiencing hypotensive metabolic ketoacidosis. I was rushed to the hospital with no blood pressure and a barely discernible pulse, with my organs shutting down. After a multitude of tests, it was determined that a mitral valve that had previously had a small regurgitation had been leaking profusely for so long that it caused the heart muscle to atrophy to the point of catastrophic cardiomyopathy (damage to the heart muscle itself). This would require more than a valve replacement—I needed a transplant!

Due to the cancer history, I had to be cancer-free for five years to be eligible for the transplant. (It had only been eighteen months at this time.) They implanted a defibrillator, and for three-and-a-half years, I existed with a central line and a bag of medication flowing 24/7; even so, my heart function was only at about 15 percent of normal. I waited, hoping that this "temporary" fix would last until I was eligible for the transplant. The hospital's BMI limit to receive a transplant was 34. I was heavier than this (well into the "obese" category), so I knew I needed to lose weight as my eligibility date got closer. My life quite literally depended on it. I took drastic measures and basically starved myself to get below the limit. (Not that I recommend this to anyone!) I lost weight and qualified for the transplant, even though my BMI was still high. I had the transplant in October 2016, weighing 175 pounds (79 kg). Transplant recipients receive numerous medications, including steroids to suppress the immune system, and many of these medicines cause weight gain and fluid retention. Steroids are notorious for raising blood sugar, so my diabetes was made even worse. I needed to take two different kinds of insulin daily.

I followed the diet recommended by the hospital dietitian (a diet recommended by the American Diabetes Association) and actually gained weight; it got up to 205 pounds (93 kg). By this time, I was post-menopausal and fighting hormonal changes. Combine that with taking medications that caused weight gain, and it was nearly impossible to lose weight. I was close to the heaviest I'd ever been in my life and feeling miserable. I was distraught that I had been given the blessing of a new heart, and I was at risk for damaging it by being overweight and having diabetes.

In 2017, I tried a commercial weight-loss program centered around counting calories. I also started exercising and lost only 14 pounds (6 kg) over six months, with no improvements in any of my health conditions. You can't blame me for feeling discouraged, and I went back to my normal way of eating, which was basically no rules at all. Later that year, I was researching fatty liver and somehow came across a video by a medical doctor who said it's possible to reverse fatty liver through diet. I was excited and asked my gastroenterologist about it. He said this was not possible. Well, I had learned from my previous health debacles that I had to be my own advocate, so I began to do more research. I went down the path from fatty liver to diabetes, to autoimmune issues, and began following a lot of doctors, nutritionists, and other health professionals on social media. I read and watched everything I could.

I learned about gut health and the negative effects of chronic inflammation. I felt like keto might be the answer for me, but I was concerned because I was a transplant patient. Someone recommended a keto-friendly doctor who told me that not only would it not be dangerous, but in fact, it would be quite beneficial. Additionally, this doctor's practice focused on peri- and post-menopausal women, so I decided he was the one for me! I had my first consultation with him in January 2019.

In the meantime, I asked all my physicians—especially my transplant cardiologist—for input. Most had not heard of keto, and some who knew about it warned me against trying it. My cardiologist said that he didn't know much about nutrition, and that if I wanted to try it, I should just stay away from anything too extreme. I was determined that I was going to do this! I enjoy a challenge, and this was the time to take action.

After I had my first consultation with the keto doctor, I was convinced this was the right thing for me. I was going to turn my life around and do this new heart justice! We agreed I should lose about 50 pounds (23 kg). I started on February 5th, 2019. I weighed 205 pounds (93 kg). My HbA1c was 7.9. I was taking two forms of insulin, three blood pressure medicines, and an antacid for acid reflux, and I was living with IBS, rosacea, psoriasis, bloating, edema, severe hot flashes, and fatigue. I couldn't lose a pound to save my life. The thought of losing 50 pounds was practically a fantasy.

It was a bit of a struggle at first, and the learning curve was steep. Everyone's low-carb experience is different. As a post-menopausal woman, I do best with a slightly lower fat intake than on a more classical ketogenic diet. I started taking my measurements early in the process as my doctor suggested, because it would help me see I was making progress even if my scale weight wasn't changing much. I'm not done yet, but here's where I am today, 11 months into my keto life: I weigh 145 pounds (66 kg). My HbA1c is 5.7. With my doctor's supervision, I've been able to stop taking both insulins, and I take only one mild medication for blood pressure. My GERD is gone, I have no bloating or edema, and my fatty liver has been reversed. My hot flashes are down to a minimum, and the psoriasis is gone. My skin is healthier, my mood is great, I have boundless energy, and all of my inflammatory markers are down, which makes everything better. I have lost 44 inches (112 cm) on my body overall—including 10 inches (25 cm) from my waist! My pants size has gone from a U.S. 18 to an 8. Some of my medical issues will never be cured, but thanks to keto and my doctor's help, the effects are minimized, and my quality of life is at an all-time high. I have never been happier or healthier. To me, this is nothing short of a miracle.

One must be cognizant that along with all the trustworthy and reliable information out there about low-carb and keto, there's also a lot of misinformation. I found many people willing to share their expertise and experiences—medical and healthcare professionals as well as regular folks like me who had had their own transformations. I am truly grateful for every blog, podcast, video, and book that people take the time to create and share with the public. I am constantly learning and growing in this journey and have adopted this as a way of life. My husband has even joined me, and he's lost 60 pounds (27 kg)! It's easier to eat this way with a supportive partner, but I would do it either way.

This way of eating and the community surrounding it gave me the knowledge, support, and the tools to save and improve my health and life. I am forever grateful. And now, I'm passing this information along to others. As I mentioned, most of my doctors were skeptical about keto, and some were flat-out against me trying it. Now that my results are undeniable, though, most of them are pleased, and my gynecologist even asked me for specifics about what I'm doing because she sees many patients who could use the assistance.

—Cheryl B., Largo, FL

CHAPTER 7

ADAPT YOUR LIFE DIET PHASE 1

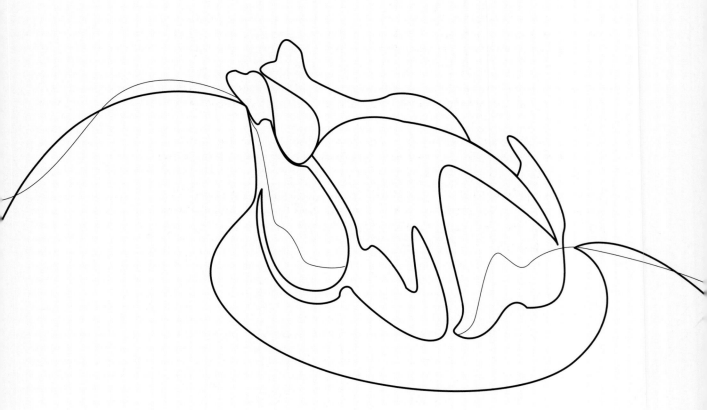

If your numbers in the table in the previous chapter led you to Phase 1 of the ADAPT Your Life Diet, *congratulations!* You're on your way to feeling better. There are just a few concepts for you to understand, and then you can put the pedal to the metal and get going. If your numbers led you to Phase 2 or Phase 3, start here and then proceed to the chapter about the appropriate phase for you.

As you'll soon see in the Phase 1 food list, Phase 1 has the lowest total carbohydrate allowance. Think of prescription drugs and over-the-counter versions. Over-the-counter drugs work, but the prescription strength options are stronger. The higher-carb approaches you'll see in Phases 2 and 3 might work for you, but the prescription strength of Phase 1 is more powerful. If your current weight or health situation points you to Phase 1, then you've probably felt unwell and run down for a long time. If you're "sick and tired of feeling sick and tired," then you don't want to mess around with something that *might* work. You want to come at things full-on and get *results*. If you're living with a lot of excess weight or you have a condition driven by high blood sugar or insulin, the most effective thing you can do is stop eating foods that raise your blood sugar and insulin the most, and that's carbohydrates.

The more generous carbohydrate allowances on Phase 2 and Phase 3 of the ADAPT Your Life Diet *might* be effective for you, but Phase 1 *will* be effective. You don't have to cross your fingers and hope for the best. I've been using Phase 1 in my practice for 20 years, and I'm presenting it to you with the confidence of the prescription drug I mentioned a minute ago: the proven success record of Phase 1 is so solid and so reliable that if the Phase 1 food list were a pharmaceutical drug, it would be approved by the FDA.

> " If you're carrying a **lot of excess weight** or have a condition driven by **high blood sugar** or **insulin**, the most effective thing you can do is **stop eating foods** that raise your blood sugar and insulin the most, and that's **carbohydrates**.

Still not sure whether ADAPT Your Life Phase 1 is right for you? If you've filled out the table in Chapter 6 and you're still uncertain which phase is best for you to start with, consider the following:

Is your quality of life limited by a medical problem, be it physical or psychological? Does your weight or a health issue interfere with your ability to participate in social activities or physical pursuits you enjoy? Or do you not have a diagnosed condition, but you know you don't feel your best? Are you tired or achy all the time, or saddled with brain fog? Do you experience mood swings that worry you or that make people around you uncomfortable? Have you felt unwell for so long that you don't even remember what it's like to feel good?

If any of these statements apply to you, I encourage you to give Phase 1 a try to see if it can correct or improve these issues.

As I mentioned in Chapter 6, even if the boxes you checked in the table pointed you to Phase 2 or Phase 3, I encourage you to read about Phase 1 and consider following the plan for some amount of time. You might resolve issues you don't even realize you have until you no longer have them. Minor things you've been living with for so long that you've come to accept them as "normal" might disappear. Just because certain things have become *common* doesn't mean they're normal. If you pop several antacids or aspirin tablets multiple times a week or your purse or briefcase could pass for a small pharmacy, give Phase 1 a try for a while even if Phase 2 or 3 seemed like the place you should start.

> "You know that old saying: If you **want something** you've **never had**, you've got to **do something** you've **never done**. *You're giving up sugar and starch, but in return you'll* **get your life back**.

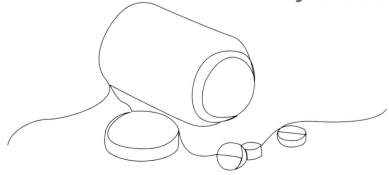

The ADAPT Your Life Diet Phase 1 Food List

This list is designed to keep your total carbohydrate intake to 20 grams or fewer per day.

If you follow the instructions in this section and consume only the foods on this list, you will not need to weigh or measure your food. Your carbohydrate intake will be 20 grams or fewer per day. You may cook or prepare the foods any way you like (grill, roast, steam, boil, fry, broil, sous vide, etc.) as long as you don't add any carbs, such as flour-based breading or batter.

See Appendix C for a handy cheat sheet of the Phase 1 food list that you can photocopy to put on your fridge or keep in your purse, briefcase, or car. I suggest taking a picture of it on your phone so you'll always have it handy.

Protein: Unlimited

Eat as much as you want of these foods until you are comfortably full:

- **Red meat:** Beef, lamb, bison, venison, elk, other wild game, organ meats
- **Pork:** Pork loin, chops, shoulder, sausage, ham, bacon, salami, ground pork, organ meats
- **Poultry:** Chicken, turkey, duck, goose, Cornish hen, quail, pheasant, other fowl, organ meats
- **Fish and shellfish:** Any finfish, including tuna, salmon, sardines, mackerel, catfish, tilapia, trout, flounder, snapper, sole, cod, etc.; shellfish and crustaceans including shrimp, scallops, crab, and lobster
- **Eggs:** Whole eggs, including yolks and whites (all poultry eggs are permitted—chicken, duck, goose, etc.)

Regarding Red Meat, Pork, and Poultry

Any and all cuts are allowed: ground meats, steaks, chops, roasts, and processed meats such as sausage, bacon, liverwurst, pepperoni, salami, deli meats (aka lunchmeats or cold cuts). Just be sure to read the labels because cured meats and deli meats may be made with sugar or brown sugar. The amount remaining in the finished product will often be negligible, but sometimes the carb content will be high for a relatively small serving. When unsure about the total amount of carbohydrate in something, opt for something more likely to be zero-carb or close to it—for example, plain roast beef or pastrami rather than brown sugar ham or honey and maple turkey breast. Regarding poultry, any cuts of chicken, turkey, duck, and other fowl are permitted: breasts, drumsticks, thighs, wings, etc. You do not need to buy lean meat or skinless poultry. You're allowed to eat the fat now—enjoy juicy steaks, fatty pork chops, and crispy chicken skin! But if you're trying to lose weight, don't add *extra* fat to meats that are already fatty.

Regarding Fish and Shellfish

Canned fish is fine (tuna, salmon, mackerel, sardines, etc.). Make sure to read labels when purchasing canned fish, though: Buy plain varieties that contain no sauces or added sugar, or stick to seasoned varieties that are very low in total carbs. Oysters, clams, and mussels are slightly higher in carbs, so use them sparingly. Avoid imitation crabmeat and other imitation seafoods because they're typically made with starchy fillers and are high in carbs.

Foods Allowed in Limited Amounts

- **Leafy greens and salad vegetables:** Up to 2 cups per day. Measure them uncooked; 2 cups is approximately the size of two fists: arugula, bok choy, cabbage (all varieties), chard, chives, endive, greens (including beet, collards, mustard, and turnip), kale, lettuce (all varieties), parsley, spinach, radicchio, radishes, scallions, and watercress. (If it's a leaf, you can eat it!)

- **Nonstarchy vegetables:** Up to 1 cup per day. Measure them uncooked; 1 cup is approximately the size of one fist: artichokes, asparagus, broccoli, Brussels sprouts, cauliflower, celery, celery root (celeriac), cucumber, eggplant (aubergine), fennel, green beans (string beans), jicama, kohlrabi, leeks, mushrooms, okra, onions, peppers (bell pepper/capsicum [note that green have fewer carbs than red, orange, or yellow], jalapeño, poblano, serrano), pumpkin, rhubarb, shallots, snow peas, sprouts (bean and alfalfa), sugar-snap peas, summer squash, tomatoes, wax beans, yellow summer squash, zucchini (courgette).

- **Cheese:** Up to 4 ounces per day. Includes hard, aged cheeses such as Swiss, cheddar, Gouda, Gruyere, Colby, and Jack, plus softer cheeses like brie, Camembert, bleu, mozzarella, goat, and cream cheese. Most cheeses are allowed on Phase 1, but be sure to read labels to check the carbohydrate total. Soft cheeses that are higher in carbs, such as cottage cheese and ricotta, are not permitted.

- **Added dairy fats:** Up to 2 tablespoons per day. Includes butter, ghee, heavy whipping cream, heavy cream, light cream (also called table cream), sour cream, and half and half.

- **Salad dressing and added oils:** Up to 2 tablespoons per day. Includes olive oil, avocado oil, sesame oil, coconut oil, canola oil, peanut oil, palm oil, other added oils.

- **Mayonnaise:** Up to 2 tablespoons per day.

- **Avocado:** Up to ½ of a fruit per day.

- **Olives:** Up to 6 per day.

- **Lemon/lime juice:** Up to 2 tablespoons per day.
- **Pickles:** Up to 2 servings per day. Choose dill or sugar-free pickles; always read labels and check for total carbs.
- **Soy sauce:** Up to 2 tablespoons per day.

Zero-Carb Snacks: Unlimited

Sugar-free gelatin, pork rinds, pepperoni slices, salami, hard-boiled eggs, low-carb jerky. (Read labels on jerky; plain/original flavors will be lower in sugar than teri-yaki, BBQ, and other flavors.) You may also snack on any of the unlimited proteins listed earlier—for example, canned tuna, deli roast beef or turkey, cold leftover chicken or bacon, etc. Cold leftover meats make great snacks!

Beverages: Unlimited Zero-Carb Beverages

Water, coffee, tea (black, green, herbal), diet soda, diet/sugar-free iced tea, zero-calorie, zero-carb sugar-free flavored drinks, zero-carb flavored seltzers or sparkling waters. Caffeinated and carbonated beverages are fine as long as they are zero-carb. Coffee and tea are unlimited but be mindful of how much cream you add if you don't drink them black.

Seasonings: Unlimited Herbs and Spices

Basil, black pepper, chili powder, cilantro, cinnamon, curry powder, dill, garam masala, garlic powder, ginger powder, nutmeg, oregano, paprika, parsley, pepper-corns, rosemary, thyme, turmeric, etc. Make sure any herbs and spices you use contain no sugar; blends or dry rubs for meat often contain sugar. (You may also use fresh garlic or ginger, but these are higher in carbs than the powdered forms, so be mindful of how much you use.)

Other Flavorings

- **Vinegar:** All varieties are unlimited except balsamic, which is higher in carbs. Use balsamic vinegar sparingly or not at all.
- **Hot sauce:** Read labels; many contain sugar. Use only unsweetened varieties.
- **Mustard:** All varieties are unlimited except honey mustard or any other variety that contains sugar or honey. Do not use sweetened mustard.
- **Salad dressings:** Read labels and include the carbs in your total for the day. Avoid obviously sweet dressings like thousand island, French, Russian, honey mustard, and raspberry vinaigrette. Stick to ranch, blue cheese, and other dressings that typically have only 1 to 2 grams of carbohydrate per serving.

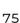

- **Salsa:** Read labels and include the carbs in your total count for the day. Avoid salsas that contain mango, corn, black beans, and anything not included in the preceding lists. Many salsas contain only tomatoes, onions, peppers, spices, and vinegar. Use these.

Have you picked up on a theme here? *Read labels and count the carbs toward your total for the day!*

Ideas for Substitutions

- **Rice:** Riced cauliflower or broccoli (available fresh or frozen in most supermarkets)
- **Noodles:** Spiral-sliced zucchini, yellow summer squash, or shirataki "miracle" noodles (available online or in the produce section of most supermarkets)
- **Milk:** Unsweetened almond milk, cashew milk, coconut milk, or other nut milk. Be sure to buy the unsweetened versions and include the carbs in your total for the day.
- **French fries:** Jicama or zucchini fries
- **Mashed potatoes:** Mashed cauliflower or celery root purée
- **Roasted potatoes or home fries:** Roasted radishes
- **Hummus:** Cauliflower or zucchini hummus
- **Bread or wraps:** Egg wraps (thin, crêpe-style), lettuce or cabbage leaves
- **Chips and dippers:** Pork rinds, cheese crisps (made from 100% cheese), cucumber or jicama slices, celery sticks, sliced raw bell pepper

A Note About Food Quality

Your food does not need to be organic, free-range, grass-fed, or pasture-raised, but I recommend that you buy the best quality food you can afford. Whether this means shopping at a local farmers market, a high-end co-op, or opting for what's on sale at your local supermarket or discount store, *as long as you stick to the food list, ADAPT Your Life Phase 1 will work for you.* See the frequently asked questions in Chapter 11 for details.

Regarding Dining Out

You will have no problem sticking to Phase 1 when ordering in restaurants or grabbing something quick while you're on the road. See Chapter 13 for tips on how to customize your order to stay within the Phase 1 carb allowance in these situations.

Sample ADAPT Your Life Phase 1 Menus

Here's what a few days on Phase 1 might look like:

- **Breakfast:** Ham and cheese omelet, coffee or tea
- **Lunch:** Bunless burger topped with bacon, grilled onions, and pickle slices; side salad with ranch dressing
- **Dinner:** Grilled salmon with roasted Brussels sprouts
- **Snacks:** Pork rinds, zero-sugar beef jerky, ADAPT Keto Bar—but remember, you might not need to snack at all!
- **Beverages:** Water, coffee, tea, sugar-free flavored beverages

- **Breakfast:** Meat and veggie breakfast hash (loose sausage with diced bell peppers, onions, and zucchini); coffee or tea
- **Lunch:** Philly cheesesteak (no roll); water or sugar-free flavored beverage
- **Dinner:** Baked pork chop with mashed cauliflower
- **Dessert:** Sugar-free gelatin topped with whipped cream
- **Snack:** Canned fish, celery and jicama sticks—plain or with blue cheese dressing or guacamole
- **Beverages:** Water, coffee, tea, sugar-free flavored beverages

- **Breakfast:** Leftover meatloaf (no breadcrumbs—yes, it's fine to have dinner food for breakfast!); coffee or tea
- **Lunch:** Antipasto plate (salami, prosciutto, other cured meats, cheese, olives, marinated artichoke hearts or mushrooms)
- **Dinner:** Chicken and broccoli casserole made with cheese and cream; side salad if desired
- **Snacks:** Deviled eggs, pepperoni
- **Beverages:** Water, coffee, tea, sugar-free flavored beverages

See Chapter 12 for additional Phase 1 meal and snack ideas.

This Is Different...Really Different!

ADAPT Your Life Phase 1 is likely very different from how you're accustomed to eating, especially if you've never tried a low-carb diet before. But that's the whole point! You're reading this because you want something different. If what you're doing now were working, you wouldn't be reading this book.

Different is the keyword here. Focus on this *diff* word rather than on the other one: *difficult*. Phase 1 might be different for you, but it doesn't need to be difficult. I've designed it to be as simple as possible, with no requirement for weighing and measuring your food or tracking and recording what you eat.

However, *simple* doesn't mean easy. Running a marathon is simple; all you have to do is put one foot in front of the other. Do that for 26.2 miles, and you'll cross the finish line. It's simple! But it sure isn't *easy*. Phase 1 is simple, but I make no promises about it being easy. For some people, it is easy. You may feel so good—maybe better than you've felt in decades—that you'll sail through this without giving a single thought to the foods that are no longer part of your life. They were making you sick, and you're glad to be rid of them. It's also possible, though, that you'll have a hard time, and I don't want to gloss over this.

Emotion-Based Eating

The Phase 1 food list is effective for normalizing appetite, but some people eat for reasons other than true, physical hunger. They eat when they're bored, lonely, tired, happy, angry, anxious, stressed out, procrastinating, mourning, celebrating, and the list goes on. If you're not in this group, great, but if you find yourself nodding here, welcome to the human race. You're in good company.

You'll find that Phase 1 helps with this to some extent. It'll be hard for you to believe until you've experienced it, but you will be hungry less often and to a lesser extent than you're used to being. You might find several hours going by when you don't think about food, and it might be the first time in your life that this has happened. If you have a long history of turning to food for reasons other than hunger, Phase 1 won't magically make these deeply ingrained behavioral patterns stop overnight, but you will hopefully struggle with them less than you did before you changed your eating habits.

A good approach to the situation is to celebrate the things you *can* eat rather than longing for the things you're going without. Remember, you may be giving up bread, pasta, potatoes, and sweets, but what you're getting in return is energy, vitality, and empowerment.

Maybe you've spent years eating dry, skinless chicken breasts. Well, now you can have a drumstick and a thigh with the delicious, crispy skin. Maybe you've shopped for the leanest pork you could find—cuts without a single visible trace of fat. Now, you can have bacon and melt-in-your-mouth prosciutto without a shred of guilt or self-recrimination, and zero worry about how long you'll need to be on the treadmill to burn it off.

Getting Started on Phase 1

One way to make this simple strategy easier is to have a family member or friend join you in this way of eating. Moral support can be helpful when sugar or starch is calling your name. Just about everyone can follow the ADAPT Your Life Diet. Even if the people in your life aren't overweight or living with any particular health issues, they can follow the plan. Remember, no one's health ever got worse when they stopped eating sugar, and this includes children. So, whether your family or friends join you in Phase 1 or they step in at Phase 2 or 3 because it's more appropriate for them, they can show support and solidarity for you by changing some of their dietary habits for the better. There are also numerous forums and websites where you can join communities of people who eat this way, but keep in mind that there are many different versions of low-carb diets. Some of them will be nothing like Phase 1, so be careful about taking advice from people following programs that are different from yours.

Getting started with Phase 1 might require an overhaul of your fridge, freezer, and cupboards. Ridding your kitchen of all sugar and starch will be easier if you live alone than if you live among family or share a kitchen with housemates. Even if you're the head cook in your household and you're the only one following the ADAPT Your Life Diet, you'll find that there will be less of a shakeup to family mealtimes than you might think. Protein and nonstarchy vegetables are appropriate for everyone, so those parts of the meal can go on everyone's plates. Simply add a portion of starch for those who want it, but leave it off your own plate. For example, cook a chuck roast with onions, celery, and radishes in your slow cooker or pressure cooker and bake some potatoes in the oven. Household members who are eating starch can have the potatoes, and those on low-carb plans can avoid them. Make meatballs with tomato sauce and a salad on the side. That's enough for people following Phase 1, and the starch eaters can have their meatballs on top of spaghetti. (Meatballs don't require breadcrumbs, but if you're nervous about using just meat and spices, put plain pork rinds in a food processor and make zero-carb "breadcrumbs" out of them.)

You may not be used to doing things this way, but it's not rocket science. You're not going to Saturn. You're still right here on Earth, and this is the same food you're already used to eating, minus the sugar and starch. For some of you, your cooking won't change much at all; all that changes is that you're skipping the sweet and starchy items. Your family members can have them if they want, but they can also join you at any phase of the ADAPT Your Life Diet. Don't forget: no one has ever died from a bread deficiency.

The Whys and Wherefores of Phase 1

Now that you've seen the Phase 1 food list and some sample menus, you probably have questions about why certain foods are allowed, whereas others are prohibited. You might also be wondering what to expect once you get started with this new way of eating. What follows are answers to the questions I hear most frequently from my patients, and some tips to make your transition into Phase 1 as smooth as possible. (Chapter 11 addresses questions about low-carb diets and the ADAPT Your Life Diet in general. Here, I present information specific to Phase 1.)

Why Is Phase 1 So Strict?

The ADAPT Your Life Phase 1 food list can be intimidating, I know. It's likely very different from your current diet. In fact, it's probably different from how you've *ever* eaten in your life! Most of all, it's different from the kind of advice you're accustomed to receiving about weight loss and overall health. But just because it's different doesn't mean it's bad or wrong. It's just a bit unfamiliar to you. In the United States, people drive on the right side of the road, but in the United Kingdom and some other parts of the world, people drive on the left side. One approach isn't better or more correct than the other; they're just different ways of doing things.

Remember, Phase 1 is the prescription-strength version of the ADAPT Your Life Diet. You *want* the most powerful and most effective strategy. You're done wasting time with things that don't work. You're done spending time, money, and emotional energy dabbling in half-measures that haven't gotten you where you want to be. This change will take some getting used to, but look at it this way: Phase 1 isn't a punishment; it's a road map to a new life—more energy, lower blood sugar, clearer skin, sharp thinking, increased mobility, improved moods, freedom from joint pain, and possibly even a better sex life. You're giving up sugar and starch, but in return, you'll get your life back.

You know that saying, "If you want something you've never had, you need to do something you've never done"? Well, if you've been saddled with poor health or excess weight for most of your life, it's time to do something different. And if you've been healthy and fit most of your life and your problems are relatively new, it's still time to do something different. There's another old saying: "What got you here won't get you there." If you followed a higher-carb diet when you were younger and perhaps more active, that diet worked for you *then*. If it's not working for you now, try a different tactic. You don't have exactly the same taste in music, clothing, or possibly even romantic partners as you did years or decades ago. Why should you follow the same diet you did back then?

Don't mourn the foods that aren't on the list for Phase 1. Instead, celebrate the foods you *can* eat. I know it's hard to imagine life without certain foods that have been part of your daily existence for as long as you can remember, but instead of looking back at those, look ahead to the future. You're going to feel so good that you won't miss the foods that were keeping you tired, achy, anxious, irritable, overweight, and on a blood sugar roller coaster you never wanted to be on. *Sayonara and good riddance!*

Who Is Phase 1 For?

ADAPT Your Life Phase 1 was designed to work for everyone who walks through my clinic door. *Everyone.* Female; male; young; not-so-young; people who are over-weight; people with obesity; people at a normal weight; those with diabetes or prediabetes, hypertension, gout, metabolic syndrome; athletes; sedentary folks; patients who are wheelchair-bound or otherwise disabled; and anyone from any walk of life, race, ethnicity, or genetic heritage. The Phase 1 approach guarantees that anyone on the highly diverse spectrum of humanity will get results. You might be able to increase your carb intake in the future and have equal success in losing weight and keeping it off, as well as managing your health conditions or keeping them in remission, but to have the most significant and quickest possible impact on the problems you're dealing with *right now*, Phase 1 is the place for you to be.

> **Missing out** on life because of your weight or your health is **restrictive**. Cutting carbs and **freeing yourself** of these things isn't restrictive; **it's liberating**.

The further away you are from your goal, the stricter the approach you need. Phase 1 is the most restrictive level of the ADAPT Your Life Diet in terms of total carbohydrate allowance because when you are very overweight or very metabolically sick, significant carb restriction is what's most effective. If you feel like the Phase 1 food list is restrictive, remember that feeling tired all the time is restrictive, too. So is having joints that ache. Brain fog. Migraines. Infertility due to PCOS. Injecting yourself with insulin for type 2 diabetes. Spending your hard-earned money on ever-larger piles of medication. Missing out on life because of your weight or your health is restrictive. Cutting carbs and freeing yourself of these things is liberating.

The strictness of Phase 1 is also its beauty and simplicity. You don't need an advanced degree in nutrition to be successful. When you keep carbs this low, you *will be* burning fat. You won't need to track your food or test whether you're burning fat, although you can if you want to. (More on this in a bit.) At the very beginning, when you're brand-new to this, it's not a bad idea to get out some measuring spoons and see what 1 tablespoon looks like, but once you have a solid concept of that, you won't need to weigh and measure your portions. My patients have jobs, families, obligations, and, frankly, just better things to do with their time than complicate their meals with apps, spreadsheets, and food scales, and you do, too. Food should be enjoyable, and you can enjoy it without math; just cut the carbs!

> "You **don't need** an advanced degree in nutrition to be **successful**. When you keep carbs this low, you *will* be **burning fat**. Food should be **enjoyable**, and you can **enjoy it** without math; just **cut the carbs**!

Aside from people who struggle with weight or metabolic issues, people who are addicted to sugar should start at Phase 1. Use your best judgment to determine whether you fall in this category; you don't need a doctor to diagnose you. If the sugar demon has its tentacles wrapped around you, you probably already know it. If you're ready to be free of this beast for good, Phase 1 is the place to start. If you're at a healthy weight and don't have any medical concerns, Phase 2 or 3 might work just fine for you, but my experience with patients has taught me it's best to take a hard stance: eliminating sweet and starchy foods from your diet is the quickest and most effective way to get that beast to retreat. If you feel like a prisoner to sugar, get rid of it completely. You don't negotiate with criminals, and you don't negotiate with sugar.

> "Are you **addicted to sugar**? If the sugar demon has its tentacles wrapped around you and you're ready to be free of it for good, **Phase 1** is the place to **start**.

Recall from earlier that starch is just a long molecule of lots of individual glucose molecules strung together. If you find that consuming starchy foods doesn't trigger any cravings for sweets, you may be able to transition to Phase 2 and possibly Phase 3 while still keeping the sugar beast far away. But it's best to start with Phase 1 for a little while so you can experience how it feels when *you* are in control, not sugar.

Phase 1 is also the best place to start if you experience low blood sugar between meals and find it difficult to go a couple of hours without snacking. If you checked the box for hypoglycemia in Chapter 6, you were pointed to Phase 1. Even if you have no medical issues and you're satisfied with your weight, hypoglycemia alone is a reason to try Phase 1. As I mentioned in Part 1, people with hypoglycemia are typically advised to eat several small meals or snacks throughout the day to "keep their blood sugar up" and prevent the plummeting lows that cause the irritability, shakiness, dizziness, nausea, light-headedness, and ravenous hunger that characterize acute hypoglycemia. But the problem isn't a lack of sugar in your diet; the problem is that the carbohydrates you ate previously triggered a large insulin response, and this overzealous insulin brought your blood sugar down too low. Eating carbohydrates every couple of hours in this scenario is like lighting several small fires and then constantly having to put them out. The solution isn't to keep dumping water on the flames; the solution is to stop lighting fires in the first place. If you have hypoglycemia but no other health concerns, then like someone who's addicted to sugar, you might be able to transition to Phase 2 or Phase 3 after following Phase 1 for a short time and learning how it feels to have steady blood sugar throughout the day. If your symptoms start to come back, you can always return to Phase 1 for a reset.

No Fruit? No Beans?!

Nope. No fruit or beans. I know this probably comes as a surprise. You might be used to thinking of these foods, especially fruit, as ideal for a healthy diet. You've probably heard, "fruits and vegetables, fruits and vegetables, fruits and vegetables," all your life! These words have gone hand-in-hand for so long that you might think they're one and the same, and that they're equally good for you. Well, for a long time, the words "artery-clogging" and "saturated fat" were inseparable, too: *arterycloggingsaturatedfat*. The same goes for "whole grains" and "heart-healthy": *hearthealthywholegrains*. Now evidence exists that shows that the experts were wrong about saturated fat (it doesn't clog your arteries), and for people with insulin resistance and a very low metabolic tolerance for carbohydrates, whole grains really aren't any better than refined grains. Both cause a large and rapid rise in blood sugar and insulin, making whole grains anything *but* heart-healthy for those individuals.

If experts were wrong about saturated fat and whole grains, they might also be wrong about those dearly beloved *fruitsandvegetables*. Think about it: The metabolic effects of fruits and vegetables—especially nonstarchy vegetables—are completely different. Even taking into account the individual variability I mentioned when I talked about the glycemic index, your blood sugar and insulin will react very differently to a pile of sautéed spinach or some roasted eggplant than they will to a fruit salad with bananas, grapes, mango, and papaya.

> "Your **blood sugar** and **insulin react** very **differently** to a pile of sautéed spinach or some roasted eggplant than they do to bananas, grapes, apples, and mango, so let's **stop saying** "fruits and vegetables" as if they're the same things.

As for beans, sometimes they're considered a source of protein, particularly for people following vegetarian or vegan diets. Beans provide protein, but the protein comes along with a big dose of carbohydrate. You can get more protein from things like beef, lamb, poultry, and fish, and you won't get the carbs. Remember, the name of the game here is *very low carb*, and a serving of beans provides more carbohydrate than it does protein.

Limited fruits and beans are included in Phase 2 of the ADAPT Your Life Diet, and a more generous selection is part of Phase 3, so it's not that these foods aren't wholesome and nutritious or that they can't be part of a healthy diet. Many people can consume these foods with no adverse effects. As I mentioned earlier, billions of people around the world consume fruit and beans while remaining slim and healthy. However, if you are living with obesity or a condition known to be driven by chronically high blood sugar or insulin, you are not one of them, and you need to limit these foods for the time being. Don't compare yourself to people who have a higher carb tolerance than you do or who have never had a metabolic illness. They are not your metabolic peers, and what works for them will likely not work for you. Phase 1 is specifically designed to induce a metabolic shift in your body away from being primarily a sugar-burner and toward being a fat-burner. How can you expect to burn fat if you keep filling your tank with carbohydrate? For you, for now, fruit and beans are best avoided.

" **Don't compare yourself** to people who have a **higher carb tolerance** than you do or who have **never had** a **metabolic illness**. They are **not** your **metabolic peers**. What works for them will likely **not work** for you.

Are Proteins and Zero-Carb Snacks Really Unlimited?

Here's what I tell my patients: Eat as much as you want of proteins and zero-carb snacks…*but I know you're not going to want much*! If you've been choking down bran cereal and skinless chicken for a decade, you can now indulge in an entire package of bacon if you like, but the novelty of that will wear off pretty quickly. The difference between Phase 1 of the ADAPT Your Life Diet and programs that require you to count calories and track grams of this and that is that you're simply not likely to overdo the Phase 1 foods. If you eat as much steak as you like, you'll probably stop after one steak, especially if it's a large one. You're not likely to go back for a second, third, or fourth steak. Try practicing "moderation" when it comes to potato chips or honey-roasted nuts, though. Good luck!

So yes, the animal proteins and zero-carb snacks are unlimited, but if you're not getting your desired results after a while, particularly with fat loss, consider keeping track of your food for a few days. Plain, unseasoned pork rinds have zero carbs, but they're not zero calories.

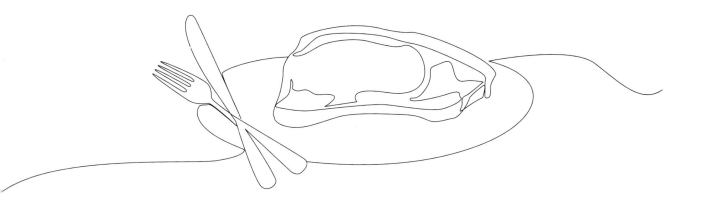

Do I Have to Eat All the Foods on the List?

No. The Phase 1 food list is what you *can* eat, not what you *must* eat. Choose what you like from the foods on the list and build your diet around those. For example, if your religious faith prohibits the consumption of pork or shellfish, omit those and eat the proteins that are appropriate for you. If you are lactose intolerant, skip the dairy products. Except for keeping carbs to 20 grams or fewer per day and not eating foods that aren't on the list, Phase 1 is entirely customizable to suit your needs and preferences. (This is true for all phases of the diet, in fact.) You can even change up the foods that are permitted in limited quantities. For example, if you don't like avocados, rather than having half an avocado, you can double your portion of cream or mayonnaise, and vice-versa.

Why Can't I Eat Whatever I Want, as Long as I Stay Under 20 Grams of Carbs?

The truth is, you probably can try eating whatever you want as long as you stay under your carb threshold, but I can't guarantee it'll work for you. The ADAPT Your Life Phase 1 food list is the road map that my patients have used to get to their destinations successfully for twenty years. If you follow this map, you'll get there, too. If you decide to go off-roading and chart your own course, though, maybe you'll get there, but maybe you won't.

You probably *could* get the results you want by eating just about anything as long as your total carb intake for the day is 20 grams or fewer, but it will likely be much more difficult than sticking to the plan laid out for Phase 1. A popular brand of chocolate chip cookie has 11 grams of carbs in one cookie—one cookie! So, two cookies and you've already met your carb limit for the day—*if* you can stop at two cookies. Maybe you can, but you'll probably be thinking about them for hours afterward and have to fight off intrusive thoughts and cravings for more. Not a chocolate fan? Salty and crispy more your thing? Nacho cheese-flavored corn chips weigh in at 18 grams of carbs for one ounce, which is about twelve chips. Twelve whole chips! No chance you'll be jonesing for more after that huge *ounce* of chips, right?

Now, have a look at the carb sources included in the Phase 1 food list. Three ounces of broccoli—triple the amount of the chip serving—has only about 7 grams of carbs, and you'd probably be okay with stopping after that amount. Even if you really like broccoli and are likely to want to eat more of it, you'd probably be able to stop at 5 or 6 ounces and not be plagued by insatiable cravings for more broccoli an hour later. The same goes for asparagus, which is even lower in carbs—only about 4 grams for more than 3 ounces by weight. You might be totally content with a few ounces of asparagus, especially if it was roasted and wrapped in bacon. The bottom line here is that you *can* experiment with including other foods in your diet as long as you keep your total carb intake very low. But compared to other carbohydrate sources, those included in the Phase 1 food list are easier to consume in controlled amounts and are less likely to provoke physical and psychological cravings for sugar or starch.

The issue of total carbs versus "net carbs" I explained in Chapter 6 is another reason it's best to stick to the foods on the list rather than constructing a diet out of anything you want as long as you stay under 20 grams of carbs a day. Food manufacturers have caught on to the popularity of low-carb diets, and they know people are cutting way back on their sugar intake. To make their products look more attractive to people who are watching their intake of sugar and other carbohydrates, these savvy salespeople have taken out some of the sugar and starch in their products and replaced them with sugar alcohols, various forms of fiber, and other fillers. If you count net carbs, you can subtract all of these carbohydrates and end up with something that looks suitable for a low-carb diet because it has a very low amount of net carbs. However, a low amount of net carbs does not automatically make something appropriate for a dietary approach like ADAPT Your Life Phase 1, where it's critically important to have a *very low* carbohydrate intake. Remember, some people are quite sensitive to certain sugar alcohols, which can induce an effect on blood sugar and insulin that might make it difficult to lose weight or improve a medical condition. For some real-world examples, numerous breads, cookies, and ice creams are available that boast low net carb counts. It's easy to polish off a whole pint of this "low-carb" ice cream or a whole tray of cookies and remain at a low net carb count, but the calories and *total carbs* can add up quickly. This is a common reason for someone to be stalled out in their fat loss, and for some people, the sugar alcohols can be an obstacle to improving their blood sugar.

Is Phase 1 a Ketogenic Diet?

Yes! I mentioned earlier that even if your current weight and health point you toward Phase 2 or Phase 3, you might choose to start with Phase 1 because you might experience certain benefits that don't come as easily with Phases 2 or 3. Some of these positive aspects result from the ketogenic aspect of Phase 1.

However, Phase 1 is more than a ketone-producing diet; it's a *fat-burning diet*. (All three phases of the ADAPT Your Life Diet help you to burn fat, but Phase 1 is the most powerful.) If you have excess weight to lose, you'll be fueled mostly by burning your stored body fat, with the rest coming from the fat in your food. If you're happy with your weight, but you're living with a medical issue driven by chronically high blood sugar or insulin, you'll derive most of your fuel from the fat in your food, which will allow you to maintain your current weight. You can generate ketones whether you're burning more of your body fat or more dietary fat, but the point of ADAPT Your Life Phase 1 is not to produce ketones. The point is to keep blood sugar and insulin controlled at healthy levels and to shift your metabolism to burning fat. The second part of that—the fat-burning—is the direct result of the first part: controlling blood sugar and insulin.

What Is Ketosis?

Ketosis is a metabolic state in which your body is burning fat. Molecules called *ketones* are produced as a by-product of burning fat, and your body can use ketones as fuel, just like it can use fat and glucose. Ketosis occurs when insulin levels are very low. There are different ways to induce ketosis, but Phase 1 does it by keeping carbohydrates very low so that blood sugar stays at a healthy low level, which means insulin does, too.

You may be wondering what makes a diet ketogenic, and that's an important question! If you've poked around keto forums and websites or flipped through keto cookbooks, you may think keto is about eating as much fat as possible—and I couldn't blame you for coming to that conclusion. A lot of the conversation is about drowning everything in butter and adding coconut oil to your coffee. *Voilà— keto magic!*

That's not accurate, though. I need to get something clear right now: What makes a diet ketogenic is the absence of carbs, not the presence of gobs of fat. The metabolic shift Phase 1 is specifically designed to induce in your body— switching you from being a carb-burner to a fat-burner—happens because you'll have very little carbohydrate coming in, not because there's a lot of fat coming in. If you could make your body burn fat just by eating more fat, you could eat five bagels, and as long as you spread enough butter and cream cheese on them, you'd be a fat-burning machine. That's not how it works, though. It's not the copious amount of fatty spreads that makes ketosis; it's the lack of the bagels.

> "What makes a **diet ketogenic** is the **absence of carbs**, not the presence of gobs of fat. Ketosis happens when **insulin levels** are **low**, and low insulin levels **don't result** from gorging on fat; they result from **not eating carbs**.

Remember: Ketosis happens when insulin levels are low. Low insulin levels don't result from gorging on fat; they result from *not eating carbs*.

Can My Body Function with So Little Carbohydrate?

Yes, absolutely! You might be concerned about this because, for most of your life, you've heard that you need carbs for energy or that your brain needs a certain amount of glucose every day, and the recommended amount is often a lot more than 20 grams. First of all, remember what "calories" are—they're units for measuring energy. And fat has 9 calories per gram whereas carbs have only 4, so if you're concerned about having enough energy, *fat* is better to eat than carbs—gram for gram, it provides more than twice as much energy. As for the brain, let's take a moment to set the record straight.

It's true that your brain needs a certain amount of glucose to function. What's important to understand is that the need for glucose is not the same as a need for carbohydrates in your diet. Your body can *make* glucose from other things. (Amino acids from protein, for example.) So even if you were to eat no carbohydrate whatsoever, your brain would have plenty of glucose available to it. If the body had no way to manufacture its own glucose, no one would survive a single day of fasting. They'd be brain dead within twenty-four hours, right? So right here, you can see the body has a way to provide the brain with glucose not only when you don't eat any carbohydrate, but even when you don't eat anything at all!

The next thing to understand about fueling your brain is that just because the brain uses a lot of glucose doesn't mean it can *only* use glucose. In fact, your brain is a champ at burning ketones. Ketones are excellent fuel for the brain, which might explain in part why people on ketogenic diets report clearer thinking and the lifting of brain fog. If your brain can use ketones for fuel, then ketones can substitute for some of the glucose it would otherwise need. Think of a hybrid car: The more electricity the car uses, the less gasoline it needs. The more ketones your brain uses, the less glucose it needs, although, at this point, scientific research has not shown that your brain can run exclusively on ketones. As far as we currently know, even on a ketogenic-style diet like ADAPT Your Life Phase 1, your brain still needs some glucose. Thanks to your body's ability to generate its glucose in-house, though, even in the complete absence of dietary carbohydrates, there'll be more than enough glucose for your brain.

> **It's true** that your **brain needs** a certain amount of **glucose** to **function**. What's important to understand is that **the need for glucose** is **not the same** as a need for **carbohydrates** in your diet. Your **body can make glucose** from other things, so even if you were to eat no carbohydrate whatsoever, **your brain** would **have plenty** of glucose available to it.

Clinical Keto Versus Commercialized Keto

As I've explained, Phase 1 is as restrictive as it is because it needs to be effective for every patient who comes to my clinic. Every single one. Some of them might be equally successful on a more liberal plan like Phase 2, but I know that Phase 1 will work for all of them without exception. People vary in their carbohydrate tolerance. Some people will be able to remain in a fat-burning state and produce ketones with a more generous carbohydrate intake, perhaps as high as 40 to 60 grams per day. But except in very rare cases with complicating factors, keeping carbs to 20 total grams or fewer will allow just about everyone to make the shift to burning fat and producing ketones.

Think of Phase 1 as *clinical* keto. Other approaches—what I would call *commercialized keto*—can work for people whose health issues are less severe, but if the table in Chapter 6 steered you to Phase 1, you don't want to mess with commercialized keto just yet. Think of clinical keto—ADAPT Your Life Phase 1—as a therapeutic strategy, and of commercialized keto as a maintenance approach. When a doctor prescribes medication or a nutritionist recommends a supplement for you, she may start out by giving you a high dose intended to be taken for a limited time. After that, she may switch you to a lower dose intended to be taken for the long term. These are usually called *therapeutic* doses and *maintenance* doses, respectively. When you're dealing with a serious, acute issue, a therapeutic approach is usually best, and a maintenance approach makes sense as the situation gets better over time. It's the same with diet.

> **Clinical keto** is **strict** but **simple**. You've **already lost** enough **years** to feeling less than your best. **Rip the bandage off all at once** and step into your new life starting ***right now***.

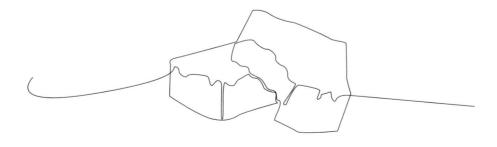

Clinical keto is strict but simple. Commercialized keto opens the door to things like almond flour brownies, coconut flour scones, low-carb cereals and granola, and other products that are marketed as "keto." These foods and products are high in fat and lower in carbs than the conventional varieties made with regular flour and sugar, but they might not be quite low *enough* in carbs to keep the metabolic benefits going for someone who is very sensitive to carbohydrate. These low-carb substitutes for higher-carb treats aren't automatically bad things. Some people can include them in their diets and do just fine, but not everyone can. I want this plan to work for everyone who's reading this right now. *Everyone*—including you. And I want it to work the first time. You've already lost enough years to feeling less than your best. Rip the bandage off all at once and step into your new life starting right now.

Commercialized keto also includes lots of things that aren't necessary and that contribute nothing meaningful to your success with this way of eating—unless you consider having a lighter wallet something meaningful. There's no shortage of products boasting claims about being essential for keto and no shortage of online "experts" specializing in fear and sensationalism who are trying to convince you that you can't do this without their pricey 14-day detox program, patented alkaline powders, or superfood cleanse.

I'm here to tell you that you *can*. You *can* be successful armed with nothing more than the ADAPT Your Life Phase 1 food list and the belief that you're worth it.

> "You can be **successful** armed with nothing more than the **ADAPT Your Life Phase 1** food list and believing that **you're worth it**.

Isn't Ketosis Dangerous?

There's a condition called *ketoacidosis*, which is dangerous, but *do not confuse this with nutritional ketosis*. Nutritional ketosis is not the same thing as ketoacidosis. Misunderstanding around this point has gotten in the way of medical and nutrition professionals recommending low-carb and ketogenic diets to the people who could benefit from them the most. It's time to clear up the confusion.

Ketoacidosis is a very rare event that happens in people with type 1 diabetes and occasionally in those with type 2. It happens when insulin doses are not properly matched to a patient's diet, or when the patient is sick, which complicates blood sugar management and changes the way their body responds to food and medications. Ketone molecules are acidic, so when they build up to very high levels in the blood, the blood can become acidic, which is a life-threatening situation. (There are also some medications used for type 2 diabetes that can induce ketoacidosis.)

However, in someone who does not have type 1 diabetes, the body has checks and balances that prevent the ketone level from approaching anything close to acidosis. In fact, in people who don't have type 1 diabetes, ketones keep their own production in check. As the ketone level starts to rise, ketone production is inhibited; ketones put the brakes on their own synthesis. One of the ways this happens is via insulin. It takes only a small amount of insulin to prevent ketones from reaching dangerously high levels. In people whose pancreas produces insulin, a rising ketone level signals the pancreas to release insulin—not a large amount as if you were eating carbs; just enough to keep the ketone level in check. In the context of a low-carb or ketogenic diet, this means your ketone level is slightly elevated, but your blood glucose is at a healthy low level, and there is no risk whatsoever that your blood will become acidic.

The situation is different for people with type 1 diabetes. Type 1 diabetes is an autoimmune condition in which the body mistakenly attacks and destroys the insulin-secreting cells in the pancreas. People with this condition produce little to no insulin, so when their ketone level rises, there's no insulin around to provide the shutoff signal. (This is one of the many reasons why people with type 1 diabetes must use insulin injections. Insulin, in and of itself, is not the enemy. It's an essential hormone! The problem many of us have is too much insulin, too often.) Also, because there's insufficient insulin, blood glucose is *high*. Usually very high, although it's possible to have ketoacidosis with normal blood glucose. This doesn't mean people with type 1 diabetes can't follow a ketogenic diet. They can; in fact, many are, with substantial improvements in their blood sugar control. (See Appendix A for details.)

The takeaway message is that the nutritional ketosis induced by a very low-carbohydrate diet, like ADAPT Your Life Phase 1, is not dangerous. The state of ketosis is what's responsible for many of the beneficial effects you'll experience following Phase 1, so you can stop fearing it and instead welcome and embrace it. Dr. Robert Atkins called nutritional ketosis "benign dietary ketosis," but controlled nutritional ketosis isn't just benign; it's *benevolent*.

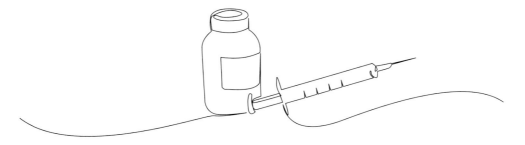

" The nutritional ketosis **induced** by **ADAPT Your Life Phase 1** is **not dangerous**. The state of **ketosis** is what's responsible for **many** of the **beneficial effects** you'll experience, so you can stop fearing it and instead welcome and embrace it. Dr. Robert Atkins called nutritional ketosis "**benign dietary ketosis**," but controlled nutritional ketosis **isn't just benign; it's benevolent**.

Doesn't Protein Affect Insulin, Too?

If you've been around low-carb and keto circles the past few years, you might have heard people recommending lower-protein diets because of the effect of protein on insulin. Protein stimulates insulin secretion, but it's different from how carbs affect this hormone. Protein induces a small, gentle rise in insulin that occurs gradually and over more time. This is a world apart from how carbohydrates—especially refined carbs—affect insulin. Refined carbs typically induce a rapid and large secretion of insulin. Think of a gentle spring breeze compared to a hurricane. Both involve wind, but they're worlds apart in order of magnitude—and magnitude of impact. The mild effect of protein on insulin is nothing to be afraid of. Insulin is a critical hormone for metabolic function and healthy life in general. You do need some insulin; what all phases of the ADAPT Your Life Diet aim to prevent is insulin being chronically high. You don't want a hurricane blowing your house down, but a gentle spring breeze across the front porch is very nice.

Whereas carbs (refined carbs, in particular) "spike" insulin—meaning, they cause a large and very rapid rise—protein induces a gradual, much lower, and *totally physiologically normal* elevation, which is nothing to be afraid of. It's a necessary effect, in fact. Remember, insulin is not a bad thing; it has many critical functions totally unrelated to blood sugar. Too much insulin, too often, is a problem, but you do need some insulin. Similarly, too much oxygen or too much water can be deadly, but that doesn't mean you should fear oxygen and water.

You probably know that insulin helps get carbs into muscle cells and other types of cells, but insulin also helps get amino acids into your cells. So if you want to benefit from the protein you're eating—to build muscle and bone; grow your hair and nails; maintain healthy skin, tendons, and ligaments, not to mention all the other things made from protein, like enzymes, certain hormones, and your immune system's antibodies—then you *want* this insulin effect. Note the word effect. This is a physiologically normal and necessary *effect*, not a pathological, harmful *spike*.

When following a low-carb or ketogenic diet—in fact, when following any of the three ADAPT Your Life Diet phases—there's no need to fear protein. Look again at the Phase 1 food list—proteins are unlimited. Scientific research has focused so much on carbs and fat and on what happens when one of these is limited. Studies that look at low-fat or low-carb diets typically keep the percentage of protein in the diet the same: either the same among the diets they're comparing or the same as what subjects were generally eating before the study. In this way, they "control" for protein while changing the percentages or total grams of carbs and fat. Protein gets the short shrift, and this has done a disservice to metabolically challenged people and people with obesity.

Protein tends to be very filling and satiating, especially when it's consumed along with the fat that occurs naturally with it. *Filling* means exactly that: It fills you up relatively quickly. *Satiating* means it keeps you full for an extended period. Think about it: If you ate a large steak or pork chop, or a plate of sausages and eggs, you'd probably feel satisfied for a while. But if you ate the same number of calories from candy, ice cream, potato chips, or cereal—the same number of calories!—you'd likely be hungry only a short time later. It's not about the calories; it's about the hormonal effects of the foods providing those calories and the feedback these hormones give to your brain and the rest of your body. The effects of protein and fat are quite different from the effects of carbohydrates (especially refined carbs).

> " It's **not** about **calories**; it's about the **hormonal effects** of the foods providing those calories and the feedback these hormones give your brain and the rest of your body. The **effects** of **protein and fat** are **very different** from the effects of **carbohydrates** (especially refined carbs).

Also, don't forget that whole-food proteins—beef, lamb, poultry, pork, eggs, fish, and shellfish—provide critical nutrients that you don't want to skimp on. Certain sweet and starchy foods provide these nutrients, too, but remember that there are no vitamins or minerals—none—that you get from high-carb foods that you can't get from low-carb foods. Forget the old advice that your protein portion should be no larger than a deck of cards. *Forget it!*

Why Are Nuts Excluded and Cheese and Avocado Limited?

You're right to wonder about this. If you've flipped through any keto cookbooks or lurked on online keto forums and groups, you've probably seen recipes for avocado chocolate pudding, sugar-free spiced nut mix, and fried cheese smothered with cheese, with a volcano of cheese melted on top. Yes, these foods are all "keto" in the sense that they're very low in carbohydrate, but they're also very high in fat, very delicious, and very easy to overdo. Nuts and cheese, especially, are common trigger foods—meaning that once you start, it's hard to stop. It's a rare person who can open a bag of roasted salted almonds or mixed nuts, have a small handful, and put the rest away. Have you seen the serving size on a bag or jar of nuts? It's typically an ounce. *One ounce! Ha!* If you can have *one ounce* of nuts and forget about the rest, you might be the world champion of willpower. For this reason, it's best to avoid nuts and seeds altogether on Phase 1, especially if you are looking to lose a large amount of weight.

Cheese is limited for the same reason: It's very calorie-dense and easy to overdo. A slice or two on a bunless burger, a couple of cubes as a snack, or some shredded cheese sprinkled on a salad or fajitas (minus the tortillas) is fine. The danger zone is when you sit down with a knife and a block of sharp cheddar or a wedge of nutty, aged Gouda. *Game over*, right? So you can have cheese, but the amount is restricted.

The reason cheese is included in a limited quantity, but nuts and seeds are excluded altogether, is that even though both are very concentrated sources of fat, the cheese is higher in protein, which gives it a slight advantage over nuts. (Some people also find cheese more filling than nuts.) As I mentioned in my earlier discussion about beans, nuts and seeds are considered sources of protein on vegetarian and vegan diets. If you look at the nutrition facts labels on containers of nuts, though, you'll see that nuts and seeds are far higher in fat than they are in protein. So, yes, nuts deliver a little bit of protein, but they pack a lot more fat. Nuts and seeds are permitted with Phases 2 and 3, so if you enjoy these foods, make it your goal to stick with Phase 1 long enough to significantly improve your health and lose the weight you're looking to lose, if any. At that point, you may be able to transition to Phase 2 and broaden your diet.

Do I Need to Count Calories?

No! That's the beauty of ADAPT Your Life Phase 1: It's so effective for regulating appetite that you will naturally settle on consuming the amount of food that's right for you. Besides, haven't you counted enough calories? If counting calories were an Olympic event, some of you reading this would have a lifetime of gold medals hanging on the wall. Put the calculators and apps away, stick to the Phase 1 food list, and enjoy your life.

However, remember that there's a reason nuts aren't included in Phase 1, and cheese, oils, and other very high-fat, calorie-dense foods are limited. It *is* possible to consume too much food energy (calories), particularly if fat loss is one of your goals. But it's harder to overdo these common trigger foods when they're specifically limited or are not part of the list at all. Stick to the list!

Phase 1 is designed to take guesswork, confusion, and complication out of the picture. High school math class is over; don't turn your dinner into a calculus assignment. You don't need apps, spreadsheets, special software, or wearable devices. You can use all those things if you want to; some people thrive on seeing the data. If you're one of them, track and monitor things to your heart's content. However, if you'd rather just enjoy your food without bringing numbers and gadgets into the picture, leave them out of it.

The ADAPT Your Life Diet—all three phases—is more about the *type* of food you eat than the amount. It's not about counting calories or measuring portions; it's about eliminating sugar and consuming other forms of carbohydrate within your tolerance level with the goals of improving your metabolic health and getting to and maintaining a healthy weight. I can't give you a precise number of calories to aim for because I don't know how many calories your body needs. Even *you* don't know how many calories your body needs. Only your body knows, and once your blood sugar and insulin levels are evened out after just a short time of following Phase 1, you'll be able to listen to those signals and trust them.

The often-parroted advice to "listen to your body" isn't a good way to go when the signals your body sends you are a product of wild highs and lows in blood sugar. You can't reason with a toddler who's having a tantrum; you have to remove them from the situation or environment so they can calm down and behave rationally. (As rationally as a toddler can, anyway.) And you can't reason with a body that's biochemically programmed to scream for sugar or starch. Once it *stops* screaming for those, though, as you'll experience on Phase 1, it's okay to start trusting your body's signals. When you're hungry, eat, and don't worry about calories as long as you're sticking to the food list and following the guidelines. Don't force yourself to go hungry because of worry about consuming too many calories. That kind of diet mentality—hunger and deprivation—is a thing of the past.

> "When you're **hungry**, **eat**, and **don't worry** about **calories** as long as you're **sticking** to the **food list and guidelines**. Don't **force** yourself to go hungry because of **worry** about **consuming** too many calories. That kind of **diet mentality**—hunger and deprivation—is a **thing of the past**.

If you're trying to lose body fat, you will indeed have to eat less than you're eating now. There's no way around that. I have some good news, though: The biochemical and hormonal changes that occur when you stick to the very low-carb guidelines of Phase 1 will help regulate your appetite to the point that you will feel satisfied with less food than you were accustomed to needing in the past. You might even find yourself skipping meals because you're just not hungry. (It's true! Even if you've never skipped a meal before. Even if you've felt like a slave to food for much of your life.) But you don't need to skip meals deliberately or limit your food intake. ADAPT Your Life Phase 1 often helps people do this naturally without even trying. On the other hand, if you find yourself feeling hungry all the time or your sugar cravings come back, revisit the Phase 1 food list to make sure you've not been straying from it inadvertently and eating more carbs than you realize.

Also, keep in mind that you don't need to consume the same amount of food every day. Your appetite will fluctuate naturally. Some days you'll feel hungrier than others, so why would you expect to consume the same amount of food or number of calories every day? I dislike calorie-counting and meal-planning apps for this reason. Should you eat the amount of food an app or a spreadsheet tells you to or the amount that your body tells you to? What if you've reached your calorie limit for the day but you're still feeling genuine hunger? Should you white-knuckle your way through and ignore this biological drive? Or what if you're completely satisfied but you're a few hundred calories under your limit for the day? Should you force yourself to eat more food even though you're not hungry? Not on the ADAPT Your Life Diet.

What If I'm Not Hungry?

Don't be surprised if, after only a few days of following Phase 1, you find you're simply not hungry. Something I've heard in my clinic many times (and never get tired of hearing) is patients telling me that, *for the first time in their lives*, they're not hungry.

If your entire life revolves around food—what you're having for your next meal, what you'll eat at your friend's party this weekend, what you'll grab at the drive-through on the way home, what you'll have for a midnight snack—Phase 1 could quite possibly be life-changing for you. If that sounds like hyperbole, be thankful that you haven't had the experience of feeling imprisoned by food, shackled to sugar cravings, unable to go even a little while without thinking about food or reaching for a fix. If it doesn't sound like an exaggeration—if it sounds like I've just described you exactly—double-check your seatbelt because Phase 1 is your fast lane to a new relationship with food.

My experience is that patients following Phase 1 sometimes skip a meal or even *forget* to eat simply because they don't feel hungry. These are people who, before Phase 1, wouldn't dare to miss a snack, let alone a meal. In a world where self-proclaimed experts have told you to eat five or six small meals a day to "keep your metabolism revving," it's a bit strange that I have to permit patients *not* to eat. Skipping a meal or two here and there will not put you in "starvation mode" and will not slow your metabolism. In fact, by keeping you in a low-insulin, fat-burning state, it may help facilitate fat loss and improvement in health conditions.

> ❝ Don't be surprised if, after only a **few days** of following **ADAPT Your Life Phase 1**, you find you're simply **not hungry**. I never get tired of hearing patients tell me that, for the first time in their lives, they're not hungry.

If you're wondering why you find yourself feeling less hungry on Phase 1, and why, all of a sudden, you're no longer thinking about "willpower and discipline" when it comes to managing your appetite and food intake, remember, it's because at the very low carb intake on Phase 1, you're already getting the fuel you need. At the cellular level, you are consuming your own stored body fat. In fact, the whole point of Phase 1, particularly when you're looking to lose a large amount of weight, is to switch you from being a carb-burner to a fat-burner. If you have health issues unrelated to your weight, the fat-burning state Phase 1 will put you into can help you maintain your weight while resolving other issues.

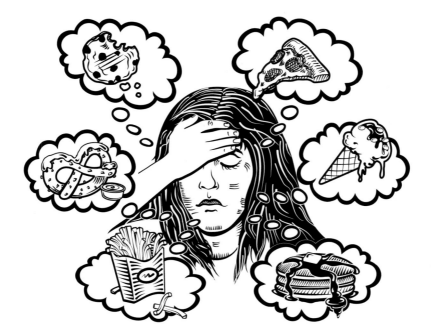

Fig 7.1: If obsessive thoughts of food have plagued you all your life, Phase 1 could be life-changing for you.

In general, the appetite regulation you'll experience through Phase 1 works through two things. First, the normalization of your blood sugar and insulin levels helps kill sugar cravings. Second, your body burning its stored fat makes you less hungry overall. When your cells are already being fed *internally*, you have less need for fuel coming in from the outside. Of course, this doesn't mean you'll never get hungry. Even when you're burning stored fat, your body still needs amino acids, essential fats, and other nutrients, and other hormones aside from insulin affect appetite. So understand that you're not doing anything wrong if you do experience hunger on Phase 1.

The difference you'll likely notice between hunger before Phase 1 and hunger while you're on the plan is that your hunger is *manageable*. It'll come on gently and gradually rather than rapidly and ravenously like it might have when you were riding the blood sugar roller coaster. The irritability, panic, and sense of urgency you might have felt if you went a while without food in your former high-carb life will be a distant memory. Instead of having to reach immediately for a snack as if it were a matter of life or death (which it truly might have felt like back then), on Phase 1, you'll be able to wait until there's an appropriate time and place—and appropriate food—to eat.

What if I *Am* Hungry?

As I've mentioned a few times, it's okay to eat when you're hungry. There's no need to deprive yourself of food or deliberately abstain from eating when you are genuinely hungry. (Remember, once you're off the blood sugar roller coaster, you can trust your hunger signals because you won't be craving sweets anymore. Sugar cravings are not indicative of true physiological hunger.)

So, when you're truly hungry, eat, but keep in mind that you don't have to eat immediately upon feeling the first very gentle hunger pang. When you're driving a long distance, do you stop to fill your gas tank every five miles? Most people don't top off as soon as there's a tiny bit of room in the tank; they go for a while on the fuel that's still left, and they fill up when the supply is much lower.

> "
> If you feel a **slight sensation** of **hunger**, you don't need to reach for a snack or have your next meal right away. Your **stored body fat** is the **fuel** that's already **in your tank**, and most people—even those who aren't overweight—have **plenty of it** to spare.

So, if you feel a slight sensation of hunger, you don't need to reach for a snack or have your next meal right away. Your stored body fat is the fuel that's already in your tank, and most people have plenty of it. Even if you're lean and aren't looking to lose any weight, you still have a supply of body fat to draw on between meals, which is exactly what your body fat is for.

If you like to live on the edge, you might be in the regular habit of driving a few miles with the gas light on. Your tank is almost empty, but you push the limits and hope you have enough to get home or to the nearest gas station. You don't need to do this with food. I'm not suggesting you wait to eat until your hunger is redlining and you're ravenous. What I *am* suggesting is that it's okay to let yourself feel a bit hungry. We are fortunate to have abundant food available all day long, all year long. Modern food production technology has made it so that droughts and other natural disasters have very little effect on the food supply. Many people have never had to go hungry because of food scarcity. In the dead of winter, you can go to a supermarket and find a bounty of tropical fruits. At the height of summer heat, you have 24/7 access to frozen desserts and ice-cold beverages. Candy and snacks are now sold at electronics stores, shoe stores, and just about everywhere else.

You are surrounded by food, which is both a blessing and a curse. You may never have gone a day without snacking, let alone deliberately skipped a meal. It's okay to let yourself feel hunger, though. Reacquaint yourself—or maybe get acquainted for the very first time—with how it feels to be hungry. Hungry, yet not uncomfortable—that's the beauty of the ADAPT Your Life Diet.

What If I Don't Need to Lose Weight?

Good question. I talk a lot about fat loss throughout this book, but the ADAPT Your Life Diet—including Phase 1—isn't solely for people who are looking to lose weight. In Part 1, I mentioned that millions of people who are content with their weight may still be afflicted with things like hypertension, gout, PCOS, mood swings, severe PMS, nonalcoholic fatty liver disease, BPH, migraines, fatigue, or other issues. The metabolic shift that happens during Phase 1 is designed to improve all of these conditions, not just help people lose weight. (In fact, the ketogenic diet was originally created in the 1920s to help children with epilepsy; it wasn't about weight loss at all.)

Phase 1 is a *fat-burning diet*. Depending on how much you eat, it can be a weight-loss diet, a weight-gain diet, or a weight-stabilizing diet. The point of this approach is to get your body into a fat-burning state. Burning fat doesn't automatically mean losing body fat. You can burn the fat on your plate or the fat on your body—this is why concentrated sources of fat, like cream and mayonnaise, are not unlimited on Phase 1 if your goal is to lose a lot of body fat. If you overdo fat from your foods, your body won't need to tap into its stored fat. Whether you lose weight, gain weight, or maintain your weight is determined by how much you eat.

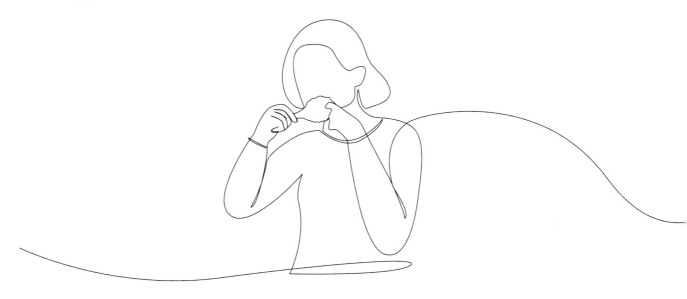

Now, you might be thinking, "Wait a minute... Doc, did you just tell me weight is determined by how much I eat? Isn't that basically saying this is all about calories? And didn't you say this isn't about counting calories?"

Allow me to clarify. This is about calories, but not in the way you think. The secret of the Phase 1 food list is that it will help to normalize your appetite to the point that you will self-adjust the amount you eat without specifically having to weigh, measure, or track your food. Counting calories implies deliberately and intentionally controlling the amount of food you eat—*limiting it*, in the case of weight loss. But as I've explained, once you're off the blood sugar and insulin roller coasters and your body is able to "eat" its own stored fat, you'll find yourself experiencing less intense hunger and less *frequent* hunger than you're accustomed to. As a result, you will likely eat less, but this will happen naturally, without deliberate effort on your part. Eating less is great if you have excess fat to lose. If you don't have excess fat to lose, your hunger will kick in to tell you it's time to eat.

> " **Phase 1 of the ADAPT Your Life Diet** isn't solely for people who are looking to lose weight. Many people who are **content** with their weight are **living with hypertension, PCOS, hypoglycemia, mood swings, severe PMS, migraines, fatigue**, or other issues. *The metabolic shift that happens during Phase 1 is designed to **improve all** of these, not just help people lose weight.*

What About Fiber?

Since Phase 1 has an upper limit of 20 total grams of carbohydrate per day and a limitation on the amount of vegetables you eat, you might be wondering where you'll get your fiber. There's no solid scientific evidence that you must consume a certain amount of fiber every day for optimal overall health or optimal digestive or gastrointestinal function. Think about it: Carnivorous animals in the wild, like lions and wolves, don't chomp down copious amounts of leafy greens every day, and they seem to have no trouble with bowel movements. I'm not saying that humans are strict carnivores with the same intestinal tracts as lions, but no one knows what the absolute minimum requirement for fiber is in a healthy human diet—if there even is one at all. The funny thing is that when you eliminate sugars and starches from your diet—cookies, cake, cereal, crackers, chips—and replace some of those carbs with spinach, zucchini, broccoli, cabbage, and other non-starchy foods, you might end up eating *more* fiber than you were before. Even better, you'll get fiber without blood sugar and insulin bombs. Bran muffins and flax-fortified cereals aren't the only ways to get fiber!

What About Constipation?

Most people don't experience constipation living within the Phase 1 carb allow-ance. However, if you think you become constipated after starting Phase 1, here are some things to keep in mind.

Constipation is not defined by the frequency of your bowel movements—that is, how *often* you go doesn't determine whether you're constipated. It's okay if you don't have a BM every day. If you had a BM daily like clockwork on a high-carb diet and you find yourself going less frequently since starting Phase 1, your fiber intake possibly *has* decreased. If you're consuming less fiber, then you have less indigestible material your body needs to get rid of, and that's fine! Nobody's going to get an award for the most bowel movements or have their tombstone engraved with the achievement that they passed the most fiber through their colon.

Consuming less fiber and having less frequent BMs doesn't mean you're con-stipated. If you only go a few times a week, but your stools are well-formed and easy to pass, you don't feel pain or have to strain to pass them, and your bowel completely empties, then you're not constipated. On the other hand, if your stools are hard or dry, you feel pain or have difficulty passing them, and you're not able to empty your bowel completely (you feel like there's more stuff still left up there), then *that's* constipation. Even if you do have a BM every day, if it's painful or incomplete or your stools are hard and dry, you're experiencing constipation.

If you're constipated and are concerned about it, you could increase your fiber intake, but eating more fiber doesn't always fix constipation. Constipation has many different causes besides inadequate fiber intake, and for some peo-ple, adding more fiber can make things *worse*. (If your colon already isn't moving waste along so well, why would you want to create more waste for it to deal with? When you have a traffic jam, the last thing you want to do is to add more cars!) Sometimes increasing your fluid intake, especially plain water, can help constipa-tion, but the most reliable remedy is to supplement with magnesium. A teaspoon of milk of magnesia at bedtime for about a week usually does the trick, or you can use magnesium citrate powder or herbal laxative teas if you prefer.

Do I Have to Measure Ketones?

No. The beauty of Phase 1 is its simplicity. If you stick to the plan as written, you will be in ketosis, so you won't need to measure. (It's possible to test for ketones so that you can be sure you're in a fat-burning state and that your carbohydrate intake is low enough that your body is generating ketones.) If you're new to the ketogenic way of eating and you've seen people on social media posting pictures of their ketone meters or read posts on keto forums and websites from people boasting about their ketone levels, you might think measuring your ketones is required. It isn't. You can measure if you want to, but your results will speak for themselves even if you never know what your ketone level is.

There are three ways to measure ketones: blood, breath, and urine. Blood testing can be cost-prohibitive for some people. The meters are inexpensive, but the test strips are pricey and can add up quickly if you test more than once a day. Breath testing is a bit more economical because although the initial expense for the breath meter is substantial, it's reusable and will last a long time. Urine testing may be the most economical, but remember that you don't need to test at all. Like I said, if you follow ADAPT Your Life Phase 1 as written, you'll be in ketosis.

If you really, really want to measure ketones, keep the following things in mind so you can do so without driving yourself crazy.

- Any level of measurable ketones is a good sign! Seeing a higher number on a blood or breath meter or a darker color on a urine test strip doesn't mean you're going to lose weight faster or that your health problem is going to be resolved more quickly.

- Your ketone level is not an intelligent, sentient being levying moral judgment upon you. It doesn't tell you whether you're a good or bad person. The only thing it tells you is whether there are ketones in your blood, breath, or urine.

I need to repeat that, because it's widely misunderstood: *Higher ketone levels in your blood, breath, or urine don't mean you're going to lose weight faster or experience more rapid improvements in your health.* If you know you're following the Phase 1 food plan strictly—no cheats, no going over 20 grams of carbs per day—and your ketone level is low, that's okay. Some people's bodies naturally produce higher ketones than others' do. A person with higher ketones isn't necessarily following the plan better or more diligently than you, and their results may not be better than yours. They just produce ketones more readily than you do. Remember: Focus on *your* journey. There are lots of other cars on the road with you, but it doesn't matter where they started or where they're going. What matters to you is where *you're* going.

I know that some people who read this will still be tempted to measure ketones. If you're one of those people, understand that ketone levels fluctuate throughout the day. Some people find they have the highest levels in the morning and lower levels later in the day, whereas others observe the opposite. Don't take one measurement at one point in time as the sole determinant of your entire day, your entire diet, and most definitely not of your self-worth. If you don't fully internalize this point, you will become very frustrated wondering why your ketone levels aren't higher, and you might be tempted to make changes to your diet that can raise your ketone level *at the expense of the results you're trying to get.* (For example, cutting back on protein and eating more fat typically raises ketone levels, but if your goal is to lose body fat, this approach can work against you.)

> ❝ **Ketone measurements** are not your **judge and jury.** They **don't determine** whether you have a **good or bad day,** and they're not a commentary on your **self-worth.** I **discourage testing** to help you avoid this frustration and disappointment. *Your **results are more important** than your ketone level.*

I generally discourage testing because I want you to avoid this kind of frustration and disappointment. Your results are far more important than your ketone level. However, there are three reasons testing can be beneficial:

- Testing is great for motivation and encouragement. Seeing ketones register in your blood, breath, or urine, even at a low level, is proof you're on the right track. It'll show you that your carb intake is low enough to keep you in a fat-burning, ketone-producing state. Urine testing can be especially helpful for this because seeing a color change on your test strip can be the virtual pat on the back you need to stick with the plan and keep going. The reagent patch on urine ketone strips is beige, and if you're passing ketones through your urine, it'll change to pink or purple depending on your level of ketones. But remember what I said: Any change is a good sign! It might be more exciting to see it change to dark purple, but even light pink is proof you're in ketosis. You can find urine ketone test strips at drugstores and supermarkets in the United States, or you can order them online.

- If you've been following ADAPT Your Life Phase 1 for several weeks or months and you're not getting the results you want, you may be consuming just a bit too many carbs for your tolerance. Not registering any ketones at all could be a sign that you're overdoing carbs. For some people, the difference between being in a ketogenic state versus not can be a matter of just a few grams. Yes, just a few grams can make that big a difference, particularly if you are especially intolerant to carbohydrates. Revisit the Phase 1 food list and make sure you're not eating anything with hidden carbs where you might not be looking for them, like in salad dressings, sauces, marinades, or breaded or battered foods when dining out. Be sure to stay under 20 total grams per day for a few days and test again to see if that does the trick.

- If you've been testing and you're in ketosis, but you're still not noticing much improvement in the issues you're dealing with, your body may require a slightly deeper level of ketosis for therapeutic effects. Earlier I said that a lower level of ketones doesn't mean you're doing something wrong. That's still true, but certain conditions might respond better to a higher level and may require a couple of tweaks and changes to the Phase 1 guidelines. If you think this applies to you, work with a keto-savvy doctor or nutritionist to help you troubleshoot to start getting the results you want. This scenario is relatively uncommon, though. Most people will feel noticeable benefits even at a low level of ketosis. (See Appendix A for finding medical professionals who are friendly to low-carb and ketogenic ways of eating.)

Why Do I Have Bad Breath?

If you've noticed that you have bad breath or a brave loved one has pointed it out to you, congratulations—you're in ketosis! The "keto breath" you're experiencing, which is sometimes described as fruity, metallic, or just plain *bad*, is the result of acetone being expressed in your breath when you exhale. Acetone is a molecule produced when you make ketones. You might not like the way it tastes, but it's a sure sign you're exactly where you want to be: burning fat. Drinking more water may help, and it's also okay to use sugar-free mints or gum. (Be mindful of the total carbs if you use several pieces, though.)

Will I Have to Stay at Phase 1 Forever?

It depends. Some people are entirely satisfied with the foods on Phase 1. They love the way eating within the Phase 1 guidelines makes them look and feel, and they have no desire to experiment with increasing their carbohydrate intake. If this describes you, that's fine. It's okay to make Phase 1 your permanent way of eating. There's no evidence that sticking with this very low carb intake for the long term is harmful. Many people choose to eat this way for the rest of their lives. Other people, however, will want to liberalize things and see how they do with a bit more carbs in their diet. I'll explain more about how to do this in the next chapter, but for now I want to give you the nutshell version.

After following Phase 1 for a while, if you're at your goal weight or close to it, or your health issues are greatly improved or perhaps even completely resolved, you can progress to Phase 2. If things take a turn in the wrong direction—you start regaining some of the weight you lost, your blood sugar is higher than you'd like it to be, or problems that were gone on Phase 1 start to come back—return to Phase 1 to recalibrate. Make Phase 1 your permanent home with only occasional visits to Phase 2. When you live in Phase 1 almost all the time, one piece of cake at a wedding or a slice of pumpkin pie at Thanksgiving isn't going to retrigger all the health problems you've gotten rid of. It's a slippery slope, though. You never *have* to visit Phase 2 if you prefer not to. You can if you want to, as long as you go right back to Phase 1 and your visits to Phase 2 are rare and short-lived.

What About Alcohol?

I'm not going to sugarcoat this: It's best to avoid alcohol completely on Phase 1. If you're looking to lose a substantial amount of weight or you're living with a serious health issue, alcohol is not your friend.

However, I know it can be a tall order to avoid alcohol, particularly when you may also be preparing to say goodbye to some of your favorite sweet and starchy foods. If being able to imbibe *on occasion* will make it easier for you to stick to Phase 1 for whatever length of time you need to, incorporate alcohol sensibly and with the least potential for interfering with the health improvements or weight loss you're seeking, and make sure to include alcohol in your carb count for the day:

- **Beer:** Stick to light beer. Most brands are 2 to 4 grams of carbs per 12-ounce (355-ml) bottle.
- **Wine:** Stick to dry reds or whites; no sweet wines or dessert wines. Count 2 grams of carbs per 5-ounce (148 ml) glass of dry red or white wine, and be realistic about the amount you're consuming. Think conservative "restaurant pours" rather than generous "home pours." You do not need to buy "keto wine." Most dry wines have very low residual sugar—sometimes as low as 2 grams for an entire liter. (And a whole bottle is less than 1 liter—not that I'm suggesting you drink that much!) Search online or consult a wine specialty store with knowledgeable employees for recommendations for wines with very low residual sugar.
- **Cocktails:** Choose zero-carb mixers, such as diet soda, diet tonic water (ask for diet tonic water; regular may be lightly sweetened), zero-carb flavored seltzers, sugar-free flavored syrups, or fruit-flavored beverages made with sugar-free powdered drink mix.

Distilled spirits (e.g., rum, vodka, gin, tequila, whiskey, bourbon) are zero-carb. The issue with cocktails on a low-carb diet isn't the alcohol; it's what the alcohol is mixed with—orange juice, pineapple juice, grenadine, sour mix, etc. Stick with drinks and mixers that will keep your cocktails zero-carb: rum and diet cola, a dry martini, rum or vodka with sugar-free lemonade, gin and diet tonic, etc.

A word of caution: Be aware that alcohol will affect you much more quickly and more strongly than it did when you were eating more carbs. Pace yourself and go slowly! You will feel the effects more severely than you're accustomed to, and you might not realize it until you've already had too much. Don't drink on an empty stomach. Always make sure you have a plan in place for safe transportation if you're drinking someplace other than your home. And remember, if you're sticking faithfully to the Phase 1 food list, but you're having a hard time losing weight, liquid calories should be the first thing to go—including alcohol. Whether it's wine, spirits, or light beer, alcoholic beverages that are very low carb are not always low calorie, and liquid calories tend not to be filling and satisfying. Many people can easily consume several drinks *in addition* to their meals for the day, which amounts to a lot more total food energy than their bodies need. Alcohol consumption is one of the most common factors that get in the way of fat loss for some people.

What About Exercise? Don't I Need Supplements? How Much Sleep Should I Get? What About Stress Management??!!

Take a breath.

No, not like that. I mean a *looong, slooow*, deep breath.

Think about how they do triage in a hospital emergency room or at a battlefield trauma center. *Triage* means assessing the situation to determine the priorities and then tackling things in a sensible order, starting with the most critical issue and working systematically down the rest of the list. Once the most important thing is identified—the most critical thing that will have the biggest effect on everything else further down the list—*that* is where you start. You address the top priority with the intervention that will yield the biggest and fastest improvement. If you're living with obesity, type 2 diabetes, or another serious issue that is severely affecting your quality of life, mobility, or physical and mental health, then right now, for you, focusing on nutrition—what you eat—will yield the biggest and fastest improvement. Nutrition is the top priority. (Read more about priorities later in this chapter in the "Priorities" section.)

I applaud you for thinking about exercise, stress management, getting better sleep, and wondering about supplements. These things are not unimportant, but remember that you're doing triage. These issues are further down your priority list. You can get to them sometime in the future after the most important thing is taken care of. In fact, you'll probably start to address them naturally once you're feeling better. Let me explain.

If you carry a lot of extra weight or you have limited mobility due to muscle or joint aches and pains, you'll likely find that a few issues get noticeably better pretty quickly. Joint pain and muscle stiffness often improve, and people notice improved energy levels within a few days or weeks of starting Phase 1—long before they've lost an amount of weight you might expect would be required to have this kind of effect. That's how powerful the metabolic shift from burning carbs to burning fat and ketones is. You'll notice positive effects *inside* your body even before you begin to see changes on the outside.

With this in mind, once you're feeling better and you have more energy, you might find yourself becoming more active without having to force it. It will come naturally. Perhaps you were very active as a kid, but the most exercise you've gotten in recent years is walking from your front door to your mailbox near the curb. Maybe you've *wanted* to be more active for a while, but your weight, body aches, low energy, or another issue has kept you on the sidelines. I can't promise you that you'll find yourself moving around more without thinking much about it, but don't be surprised if it does happen within just a short time of starting ADAPT Your Life Phase 1. You might take the stairs at work instead of waiting for the notoriously slow elevator. Maybe you'll take the first parking space you see even if you're normally in the habit of driving around until one frees up as close to the store as possible. Maybe you'll do two loops around the block while walking your dog instead of just one. Not everyone loves to work up a sweat on a treadmill or trail or to get on a bike or into a swimming pool, but if you do enjoy those kinds of deliberate exercise and you've been unable to do them for a while, Phase 1 might help you get back to them sooner than you think.

To be clear: If exercise is already a regular part of your life, don't stop! In no way do I mean to discourage you from exercising or participating in physical activities you enjoy. I'm only saying that if you don't currently exercise, Phase 1 will still be effective for you, and you don't need to feel guilty for not being more active. I've had numerous patients in wheelchairs or who were otherwise disabled and *couldn't* exercise, and Phase 1 worked for them just as well as for everyone else. Being unable to exercise due to limited mobility or low energy will not be an obstacle to your success with this way of eating. What's responsible for improving the conditions you're living with are consistently lower blood sugar and insulin levels, and exercise is not required to achieve these.

Regarding sleep and stress, no one's health ever got worse when they got more sleep and learned to relax. However, if your current weight or health points you to Phase 1, addressing these issues is less critical than getting your diet squared away. Plus, you might notice your sleep naturally improves once you're off the blood sugar roller coaster and your body has adapted to running on fat rather than sugar. You may find that you fall asleep more easily and that you stay asleep through the night. (Sudden low blood sugar is a common reason for people to wake in the middle of the night.) If your excess weight interferes with your airway and you have obstructive sleep apnea that prevents you from getting good quality sleep, this condition may improve over time as you lose weight. Of course, not everyone with sleep apnea is overweight. If you have sleep apnea but excess weight isn't an issue for you, your condition may still improve once your metabolism is primed differently. In the meantime, if you know your sleep quantity or quality isn't so great, that's all the more reason to hunker down and be strict with the diet.

As for stress, I certainly encourage incorporating strategies into your life that can help you reframe difficult circumstances you're in or that give you some quiet time to recharge if you need it. However, in your triage situation, other issues have a bigger negative effect on your life than stress. Besides, running your body on fat and ketones rather than sugar might have a positive effect on your ability to manage stress, just as it may have a positive effect on your sleep habits. A multitude of factors plays into your ability to be emotionally resilient and remain calm in the face of stress—childhood experiences, a support system of friends and family, financial resources, etc. For some people, wild ups and downs in blood sugar can show themselves as wild ups and downs in mood and in the ability to have appropriate reactions to different situations. When your body and brain have a steady supply of fuel all the time in the form of fats and ketones, you may find yourself staying calm in circumstances that in the past would have triggered anxiety, fear, anger, or another strong emotion.

Plus, when you shift your diet away from nutrient-poor refined carbs and junk foods and consume more nutrient-rich foods like beef, pork, seafood, poultry, and green vegetables, you will likely increase your intake of vitamins and minerals that are required to synthesize various neurotransmitters and other compounds that help regulate how your body and mind respond to stress—things like serotonin, dopamine, and GABA—"feel-good" molecules that support a positive mental outlook or promote internal calm.

In terms of supplements, if your doctor has identified that you're low in a specific nutrient, then taking supplements or eating more foods that are high in that nutrient can be beneficial. But most of my patients do just fine without supplements. Remember what I said in Chapter 2: When you consume sugar, it increases your need for certain nutrients so you can properly metabolize the sugar. When you stop eating sugar, you don't need those extra amounts. Plus, there are compounds in grains and beans that interfere with the absorption of certain minerals and the proper breakdown and digestion of protein. Because you won't be eating any grains or beans on Phase 1, you may absorb more of the nutrients from the foods you do consume. If you'd like to take a multivitamin for peace of mind, that's fine, but it's not required.

Can It Really Be This Simple? *Really*?

Yes, really. You may have heard approaches like the ADAPT Your Life Diet called *lazy* keto or *dirty* keto. I prefer to think of it as *simple* keto. *Straightforward* keto. *Uncomplicated* keto. Keto for normal people in the real world, with busy lives, responsibilities and commitments, budget constraints, and a desire for something that works without requiring a PhD in physiology or a total overhaul of their lives to accommodate grocery shopping and meal preparation. You can keep your meals simple and enjoy your food without the math; just keep the total carbs lower than 20 grams a day. Actually, you don't even need to worry about counting the 20 grams: if you stick to the Phase 1 food list and follow the guidelines, you'll be exactly where you need to be.

> " You may have heard this approach called *lazy* **keto** or *dirty* **keto**. I prefer to think of it as **simple keto**. *Uncomplicated* keto. Keto for normal people in the **real world**.

Food purists and people with a judgmental streak use "dirty" and "lazy" keto as derogatory terms. They would rather people make all condiments from scratch, never use artificial sweeteners, and eat only grass-fed meats, organic produce, eggs from free-range hens, and butter from cows raised on fast-growing spring grass. There's nothing wrong with that approach if you can afford these things in terms of both time and money, but there's also nothing wrong—*absolutely nothing*—with the simple, straightforward ADAPT Your Life Phase 1 approach with a twenty-year track record of clinical success. And Phase 1's simple, straightforward blueprint allows for diet soda, string cheese from a gas station, store-bought salad dressings, hard-boiled eggs from an airport food stand, and other conveniences that make the plan easy to stick to in the real world for the long term. Success is more important than perfection. I have yet to see a randomized clinical trial proving that filet mignon from a grass-fed steer raises blood sugar less than a fast-food hamburger patty without the bun.

> " Success is **more important** than perfection. There has yet to be a randomized clinical trial **proving** that filet mignon from a grass-fed steer **raises blood sugar less** than a fast-food hamburger patty without the bun.

Unique Benefits of Phase 1

I mentioned that even if your results from the exercise in Chapter 6 pointed you toward ADAPT Your Life Phase 2 or Phase 3, you might choose to start with Phase 1 for a while. This is because there are effects you'll experience in a ketogenic state that you might not experience at a higher level of carb intake. If you're already healthy, lean, and very active, you'll probably experience ketosis at a higher level of carbohydrate intake, so you might not need to be at Phase 1. If you're not carrying a lot of excess body fat and you're not dealing with any specific medical issues, you might be able to maintain nutritional ketosis eating the more generous carb allowance of Phase 2. And if you're especially lean and athletic, with a low body fat percentage and a lot of muscle mass, you might even occasionally be in ketosis while following Phase 3. But if you stay at or under the 20-gram total daily carbohydrate allotment of Phase 1, you are certain to be in ketosis, so if you want to be sure you'll experience the positive effects that come from this, start here. If you're already healthy and fit, you'll be able to transition to Phase 2 and possibly Phase 3 more quickly than someone who starts at Phase 1 due to obesity, diabetes, or another serious concern.

Here are some of the positive things you may experience while following Phase 1 of the ADAPT Your Life Diet apart from fat loss:

- Sharp, clear thinking (bye-bye, brain fog!)
- Disappearance of sugar cravings
- Substantial improvement or total resolution of heartburn/acid reflux
- Greater physical energy
- Improved mood stability and mental outlook
- Improvement in joint pain and stiffness
- Decreased water retention and bloating
- Clearer skin
- Increased libido
- For women, lessening of menstrual cramps; less severe PMS
- For men, improved erectile function
- No more feeling "hangry"
- Less hunger; well-controlled appetite; ability to go several hours comfortably without eating

Of course, you'll experience other beneficial effects from Phase 1—critically important things like lower blood sugar and insulin levels, improved blood pressure, and a healthier lipid profile (cholesterol and triglycerides)—but if you follow the phase of the ADAPT Your Life Diet that's right for you, you'll maintain these aspects of good metabolic health on Phases 2 or 3 as well.

Let's talk about the last point on the list. You won't get hungry between meals because your body already has access to fuel. When your carbohydrate intake is this low, your insulin level will be low most of the time, so your stored body fat can be released more easily and be burned as fuel in other parts of your body. (Remember that blocking the release of stored fat is one of insulin's jobs apart from lowering blood sugar.) That's what body fat is for, in fact: it's stored fuel to keep you nourished and energized when you don't have food coming in.

Within just a few days of starting Phase 1, you'll find that you can easily go several hours without eating, even if you have a long history of needing to snack throughout the day or maybe even being *afraid* to skip a meal. The reason you'll be able to be comfortable without eating for a longer period is because, at the cellular level, you are getting fuel from your stored body fat.

A Word About Fat Loss

ADAPT Your Life Phase 1 is the strategy that will result in the fastest and most effective fat loss. The more excess body fat you're carrying, the more quickly it will come off, at least at first. So the closer you are to your goal weight when you start, the longer it might take for those last few pounds to pack their bags and leave. Younger people tend to lose weight faster than older folks, and men typically lose faster than women. Fair? No. Typical? Yes. Remember what I said about the long road trip you're taking: Don't compare your route to anyone else's. If someone in your life—a family member, friend, or coworker—is following the ADAPT Your Life Diet with you and is losing fat more quickly than you are, celebrate how well they're doing, trust the process, and know that you're doing just fine, too. *Slow fat loss is still fat loss.*

I recommend weighing yourself no more than once a week. If you currently weigh yourself daily, try to get out of that habit. It can be psychologically self-destructive and also misleading in terms of the progress you're making. If you feel that weighing yourself every day keeps you accountable to yourself, it's okay to keep doing it, but understand that small fluctuations in your scale weight are normal. These fluctuations in weight are not necessarily changes in *body fat*. Don't be alarmed by a rise of one or two pounds if you know you're sticking faithfully to the food list. Many factors affect scale weight, especially for women. Humidity, water retention, hormonal fluctuations, and even air travel can cause a small increase in weight. And a good bowel movement can cause a noticeable decrease, of course.

> **"** I **recommend** weighing yourself no more than **once a week**. If you weigh yourself every day, **try to get out** of that **habit**. It can be psychologically **self-destructive** and also misleading in terms of the progress you're making.

The point is, these small ups and downs aren't usually changes in body fat; they're fluctuations in water, and they're *totally normal*. If you live and die by the scale, these day-to-day blips will drive you bonkers. If you hit a red light on your trip, you don't just give up and go home. You wait for the light to turn green, and you continue. What matters is the long term, which is why I suggest weighing yourself only once a week. Once every two weeks might be even better—if you choose to weigh yourself at all. Regardless of whether you see the scale going up or down on any given day, take it for what it is: general evidence of how the way you've been implementing Phase 1 is working for you. Your scale weight is *not* a commentary about whether you are worthy as a human being or you deserve self-respect.

> **"** Whether you see the scale going up or down on any given day, **take it for what it is**: feedback about **how Phase 1 is working for you**. Your scale weight is **not a commentary** about your **worth as a human being** or whether you deserve self-respect.

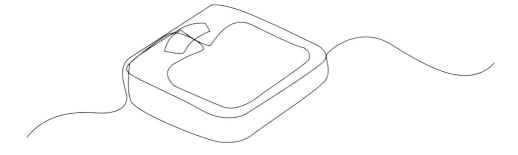

Consider ditching the scale altogether. A tape measure is a better gauge of how your body is changing because it's not uncommon for your scale weight to stay the same while your shape and size are changing. You could be losing inches even if you're not losing pounds, so taking your measurements can sometimes be a better way to track your progress, and assessing how your clothing fits is even better than that. It's not uncommon for a woman's scale weight to stay the same while she goes down a dress size. Don't let the scale play head games with you!

You will likely lose several pounds very quickly when you're just starting with Phase 1, which can be highly encouraging and help keep you motivated to stay on plan. Be prepared for the quick initial weight loss to slow down, though—sometimes as soon as the third week or so. High insulin levels cause the body to retain water—several pounds' worth in some cases. When you cut way back on carbohydrates, and your insulin level stays low most of the time, your body releases this excess water fairly early in the journey.

Despite this, don't believe what you've heard about the weight you lose on low-carb diets being *all* water weight. It's not true! Your body gets rid of excess fluid very quickly during the initial adaptation, but once the extra water is gone, you'll start shedding body fat. Twenty years of helping patients with Phase 1— some of whom have lost more than 200 pounds—tells me it's definitely not all water. And who says losing water weight is a bad thing, anyway? If chronically high insulin has caused your body to hang onto all that extra water for years, and if this fluid retention is causing problems such as hypertension or swollen legs and ankles, then it's a great thing to be rid of it.

Priorities

Earlier I talked about triage and prioritizing the most critical issue that's affecting your health, and I want to revisit that idea. Let me explain it in a simple way that will help it all make sense.

Think of your body as a sound modulator—the kind they use in a recording studio to make songs sound the best they can be. Professional sound technicians tinker with the dials and switches to adjust the bass, treble, background noise; modulate different sound frequencies; and work their magic on all kinds of other aspects to have something sound *just right*. In an ideal scenario, you would be able to do this with your health—tackle everything all at once and adjust things until every possible aspect was absolutely perfect. But what if you're not living in this ideal situation? What if even the mere *thought* of having to tackle everything at the same time feels impossible? The good news is that you don't have to.

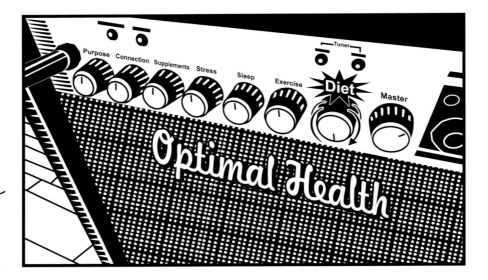

Fig 7.2: When you're just getting started, you only need to focus on one dial: your diet.

Let's say your modulator has seven dials:

1. Diet/nutrition
2. Exercise/physical activity
3. Sleep
4. Stress management
5. Supplements
6. Social relationships, human connection
7. Fulfilling work, a purpose in life

If you're starting with ADAPT Your Life Phase 1 owing to a serious medical condition or because you want to lose a significant amount of weight, then right now, your diet dial should be turned up all the way, and you can keep the other dials set to low. The other dials are *there*, and you're not ignoring them completely, but for now, all your efforts should be focused on maximizing the effects of this one dial. Worrying about the others will only distract you from your primary mission: diet. For some of you, Phase 1 will be such a big change from how you're accustomed to eating that you'll *have to* focus all your attention on the food for a while. For others, who might be a little more familiar with low-carb or ketogenic diets, it's still a good idea to get back to the basics for a while and master Phase 1 so that when the time comes to start looking at the other dials, your diet will be second nature, and you'll hardly have to think about it at all.

> **It's good** to have **sleep, exercise, supplements,** and **stress management** on your radar, but for now, **keep them** where they belong on that radar screen: in the **periphery**. Right now, **your diet is front** and **center**, and your diet is what you should **focus on**.

To take the music analogy one step further, think about learning to play a musical instrument. When you're brand-new to a musical instrument—a saxophone, let's say—you have to understand the basics before you can move on to advanced techniques. For example, you have to learn how to hold the instrument properly and where to put your hands so that your fingers fall on the right keys. Professional musicians use special techniques to make beautiful vibrato sounds or guttural growls for effect. You can learn those things sometime down the line, but as a beginner, you don't even think about them. You don't worry about what you'll wear to your recital at Carnegie Hall in twenty years. You think only about holding the instrument properly, positioning your mouth on the mouthpiece, and trying to produce *some kind of sound*.

You're just getting started on your journey to better health. For some of you, it will be a relatively short journey before you're able to move on to Phase 2 if you choose to. For others, it will be a slower process. Regardless of the length of the road ahead, what matters is where you are *now*. If you're driving from New York City to Seattle, it'll take you a few days and a few thousand miles to get there. On the day you leave New York, it would be silly to check the traffic report in greater Seattle because you won't be there for quite a while. It's more important for you to know the traffic situation in your immediate area—the thing that affects you most in the here and now.

You are right to have sleep, exercise, supplements, and stress management on your radar, but for now, keep them where they belong on that radar screen: off to the side, in the far periphery. Right now, your diet is front and center, and your diet is what you should focus on. For some of you, beginning to think about these other aspects of physical and mental health will happen naturally as you feel better *because of* the dedicated focus on diet you're starting with.

Special Considerations for Phase 1 of the ADAPT Your Life Diet

The way you'll be eating on Phase 1 might be a dramatic change from how you've been accustomed to eating for most of your life. Your body will respond to this change very quickly, and there are a few things you need to be aware of before starting so that your transition will be as smooth and pleasant as possible.

Medication

If you're taking medication for type 2 or type 1 diabetes (including insulin) or high blood pressure, you must be supervised by a medical professional who can help you adjust your medications safely as you start Phase 1. Do not do this on your own. Phase 1 is so powerful and works so rapidly that your medications may become too strong on *the first day*, and you will be overmedicated if your doses aren't adjusted. The diet will begin to improve your metabolic health very quickly, and your body will be working so differently that you may not need the same doses of medication you required when you were eating a lot more carbohydrate. Combining the natural healing effects of the diet with your medication can lead to side effects you can avoid by working with a trained medical professional who can guide you in adjusting the meds. Understand that the potential side effects (low blood sugar, low blood pressure, dizziness, light-headedness, fatigue, rapid heart rate) are not from the diet; they're coming from the combination of the diet with a dose of medication that may now be too high for you. In fact, Phase 1 works so quickly and is so powerful that your body will respond almost immediately to the removal of sugar and starch from your diet. So it's best to find a supportive medical professional to evaluate you before you even start this program. (See Appendix A to search for someone in your local area.)

Keto Flu

If you know anyone following a ketogenic or very low-carb diet, or even if you've just lurked on keto-oriented social media sites, you might have come across the term *keto flu*. The dreaded keto flu! I wish this phrase didn't exist and that instead it was called what it actually is: "The very brief adjustment period that most people sail through with no problems whatsoever but that causes a few people to experience some unpleasant but transient issues, all of which are well worth it to reclaim the vitality waiting for them on the other side." That's a real mouthful, though, so to keep things simple, I'll go with the crowd and just call it keto flu.

Going from a high-carb diet to an extremely low-carb diet cold turkey can be a shock to your body. (Even though cold turkey has no carbs...*ba-dump-tss!*) Most people have no problems making the transition, but some people experience a few issues, most of which are related to rapid fluctuations in electrolytes, especially sodium. Things you might experience include headaches (possibly severe), dizziness, light-headedness, low energy, nausea, or constipation.

Please do not be alarmed or discouraged. You'll get through it, and once you do, you'll feel much better. The worst will pass in just a few days, and it's a small price to pay to start fueling your body on fat. Here are some tips to help make the transition smoother:

- **Hydration:** Drink plenty of water. You might feel a little dehydrated because of the large amount of water your body will let go of in the first few days. (Very low-carb diets are natural diuretics—they help your body release excess water.) There's no exact amount of water you need to aim for. Drink according to thirst.

- **Headache, fatigue, dizziness:** These symptoms are most often caused by inadequate sodium. As I mentioned when I discussed hypertension in Part 1, very low-carb diets like Phase 1 change the way your kidneys hold on to sodium. When your insulin level is low, your body flushes out sodium, and you need to replace it. Sodium is an essential mineral, and you might be consuming significantly less of it on Phase 1 than you were previously. Packaged carbohydrate-rich foods are often loaded with salt as a preservative, and you've eliminated these from your diet. Don't be afraid to salt your food now. When you're on a very low-carb diet, you need more sodium, so salt your food liberally or drink one or two servings of broth made from bouillon cubes. (If you make homemade broth or stock, be sure to salt it generously. By itself, broth is not a natural source of sodium.) Any kind of salt is fine. If you prefer gourmet-style pink, gray, or black unrefined salts, go for those, but regular table salt is fine, too. What your body needs is the sodium, and that's found in all forms of salt. Do not follow a low-sodium diet unless prescribed by your physician.

- **Leg or muscle cramps:** With the rapid loss of water from your body, you'll lose some minerals, too. Certain minerals are important for muscle contraction and relaxation, and imbalances or insufficiencies in these minerals can sometimes result in leg cramps, particularly at night. If you're conscientious about getting enough sodium and are still having leg cramps, try taking supplemental magnesium or potassium to see if the cramps diminish. Again, I recommend a teaspoon of milk of magnesia at bedtime for a week, but other forms of magnesium, such as magnesium glycinate or magnesium malate, are effective, too. (If you have a heart condition, do not supplement without medical supervision.)

- **Constipation:** Remember what I said earlier—not having a daily bowel movement doesn't mean you're constipated. If your stools are hard and dry or difficult and painful to pass, *that's* constipation. If you're experiencing these issues, supplemental magnesium is effective. I recommend a teaspoon of milk of magnesia at bedtime for a week, magnesium citrate powder, or laxative herbal teas.

Most people won't have any trouble at all while their bodies adjust to ADAPT Your Life Phase 1. If you're concerned about the possibility, though, consider starting the program around your work schedule or social calendar. For example, if you work a Monday-to-Friday job, make Thursday or Friday your first day of Phase 1 so that if you experience some of the keto flu symptoms, they're more likely to occur on the weekend when you can be home and don't need to be your best. Your body has about 24 to 48 hours' worth of stored carbohydrate to use before you start transitioning to burning more fat and producing ketones, so you're unlikely to feel any difference on the first day. The second and third days are when you might start noticing some issues, so plan accordingly for your professional and social obligations.

Please also keep in mind what I said earlier about medication. Some of the symptoms of keto flu overlap with those of being overmedicated with drugs for high blood pressure or diabetes. Low blood sugar or low blood pressure can result in dizziness, light-headedness, nausea, sweating, a rapid heart rate, irritability, confusion, and, in extreme cases, even passing out. Do not mistake garden-variety keto flu with signs that your medication is too powerful and needs to be adjusted. *Work with a doctor before you start Phase 1* if you are taking medication for your blood pressure or blood sugar.

> **ADAPT Your Life Phase 1** isn't a **prison**. On the contrary, it can mean freedom for you: *freedom* from sugar cravings, from joint pain, from acid reflux, migraines, mood swings, and brain fog. Freedom from limited mobility that was restricting your ability to enjoy life. **Phase 1 isn't a punishment**; it's **a privilege**.

Transitioning from Phase 1 to Phase 2 of the ADAPT Your Life Diet

How will you know when it's time to transition from Phase 1 to Phase 2, or *if* you can?

Let's start with where you are. Remember what I said earlier: What got you here won't get you where you want to be. So, where are you right now? If you started with Phase 1 because of obesity, type 2 diabetes, PCOS, nonalcoholic fatty liver, or another serious issue, the shift to Phase 2 will take time. You won't speed through Phase 1 in days or weeks; you'll progress through it steadily over months or possibly years, depending on your weight and health status when you start. The more excess weight you're carrying and the more severe and numerous the health issues you're living with, the longer you will likely spend on Phase 1. Don't be discouraged: Phase 1 isn't a prison. On the contrary, it can mean *freedom* for you: freedom from limited mobility that was restricting your ability to enjoy life. Freedom from sugar cravings, joint pain, acid reflux, migraines, mood swings, and brain fog. ADAPT Your Life Phase 1 isn't a punishment; it's a privilege.

But let's say you've followed Phase 1 for a while. You've lost weight, you're feeling better, and various medical issues have been put into remission. *What now?* Is it time to transition to Phase 2, and if so, how do you do this?

One indicator is you're at your goal weight or close to it. You'll also know based on how you feel inside—your energy levels, mood, cognition, libido, etc. Beyond these factors, for objective proof that things are getting better, your doctor can help with measuring your fasting glucose, hemoglobin A1c, insulin, blood pressure, triglycerides, and other key health markers. If everything has gone in a good direction and you're satisfied with the progress you've made, you have two options: stay with Phase 1 indefinitely or transition to Phase 2.

If you've reached your goal weight but would prefer to stay on Phase 1, stick to the foods on the list but increase the total amount of food you're consuming so you maintain your new lower weight and do not lose further body fat. It's more likely, however, that you will opt to expand your diet and transition to Phase 2. Chapter 8 will explain how to do this.

Where to Go for Help

Still not sure if Phase 1 is right for you? Worried about making this kind of change on your own? Do you do best having other people on the same path so you can check in with them for support and accountability? Visit the ADAPT Your Life website (www.adaptyourlife.com) for educational resources to help to reach your goals. See Appendix B for details.

Fibromyalgia and Limited Mobility to Long Walks and Loving Life

"I didn't feel the need to obsess about ketone levels. What matters is that I'm happy with my results."

I am 42 years old, and I'm originally British but have lived in western Germany for the last nine years. I've been living with PCOS for more than twenty years and have taken a commonly prescribed drug for it for most of that time. Having PCOS means that I have facial hair, and my menstrual periods disappear unless I take birth control pills. I have tried to conceive in the past and barely managed to ovulate even with fertility drugs. In addition to the PCOS, I was diagnosed with fibromyalgia in my thirties, although I believe I'd had it for some years before then. I suffered with joint pain best described as a burning ache, not to mention crippling overall exhaustion. As you can imagine, at times it felt like I might as well not bother getting out of bed. Also, every now and then, if I had overexerted myself physically, my legs would just give out and not work anymore. When I went on holiday and did more walking than usual, I would have a folding walking stick on hand. I've been given many medications over the years, none of which helped much, and a few which made matters worse.

In my forties, I was diagnosed with two prolapsed discs and arthritis in my big toes. I also have knees that crunch and thumbs that stiffen in winter—issues that no doctor has been able to identify yet. My blood pressure has always been high, and I have been medicated accordingly.

Over the last few years I had moments where I've felt a bit weak and disoriented. My husband eventually figured out what this meant: hypoglycemia. He would rapidly steer me toward food, and then I'd be fine again. On one instance when this happened, I was with my mum, who has type 2 diabetes. Since these episodes didn't seem quite right, and most of the females in my family have type 2 diabetes, she urged me to get my blood checked. It turns out I had prediabetes. I reported back to Mum, and she told me about a diet her doctor had told her to go on—a low-carb diet—and how well she felt on it. I searched online for information about low-carb diets and diabetes. I watched and watched, and decided to give it a go.

I started in January 2019. To be honest, I was excited about it but also expected it to be like the other diets I had tried: I might lose a little bit of weight in the short term after the holidays, but that would be it. I thought I was already following a healthy diet—I always bought everything whole grain, didn't eat too much fat or salt, and I cooked from fresh every day.

I began by tracking everything. I had learned the difference between low-carb and keto and opted for strict keto to start. I gave up all the carbs and started to eat the keto way. In the beginning, I felt awful, but that eased quickly. As a couple, my husband and I both changed our eating habits. My husband is still a carb eater, but he eats a lot lower-carb than he used to. This works just fine for him; he's lost 10 kilos (22 pounds) without even trying that hard! For me, the weight started to shift a little, and I also took my measurements. I had heard the scale doesn't always tell the truth when your body is changing—it can be misleading if your weight doesn't change much, even if you're losing inches or centimeters. I recommend doing both—weigh yourself and take measurements.

I tracked all my food obsessively for the first few months, but it was soon clear to me that even if I did slip up a bit, as long as it was a whole food and I got right back on plan, it didn't massively impact my weight loss. I have never used a ketone meter or the urine strips. I was seeing regular progress, so I didn't feel the need to obsess about ketone levels. Seeing people on social media get so worried and frustrated because the strips showed the wrong color or a low level seemed self-punishing. I am probably dipping in and out of ketosis, but since I don't test, I can't be sure. What matters is that I'm happy with my results.

I do not do keto baking. I experimented with a few things and found I was just re-placing some of my old food habits with keto-friendly versions, so I stopped most of that with occasional exceptions. As my husband and I progressed, our physical stamina im-proved, and we now regularly walk 15 kilometers (9 miles) or so on a weekend, whereas before I couldn't have managed 5 kilometers (3 miles), or if I did, I'd be so exhausted that I was incapable of doing anything else for the rest of the day. We now walk into town (a forty-five-minute walk), whereas before we would've taken a bus. We go to the gym together and root each other on.

As I write this, it's just over one year after I started keto. I've lost 28 kilos (61 pounds). I've learned that I am an addict with regard to sugar and white carbs, and I simply must stay away from them. I avoid them now—not really from this emotional perspective, but because they honestly don't taste good to me anymore. I've been able to stop my PCOS medications, and the PCOS has improved to the point that I now ovu-late and have periods naturally, and the facial hair is starting to thin a little. I'm taking half my original dose of blood pressure medicine, my HbA1c is in the normal range, and my fibromyalgia is almost nonexistent. It flares up a little if I'm sick, but it's quiet most of the time. I used to need a nap every afternoon, and that's now a thing of the past. I can tie my own shoelaces without holding my breath—don't underestimate this accomplish-ment for someone with a history of being overweight.

Keto and low-carb social media can be fantastic resources, but many experts say different things about fiber, net carbs, fasting, calories, and all sort of other issues. Ultimately, my biggest lesson of this year was to listen to what my body is telling me. Listen to what yours tells you because you are the person who knows yourself best.

—Gayle H., Bonn, Germany

CHAPTER 8

ADAPT YOUR LIFE DIET PHASE 2

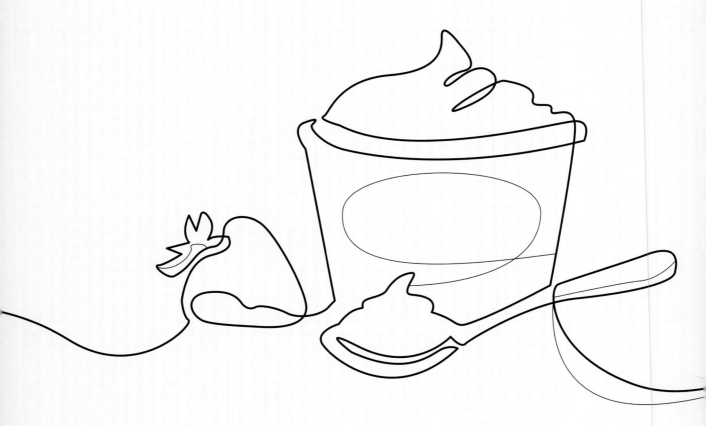

If the table in Chapter 6 pointed you toward Phase 2 of the ADAPT Your Life Diet, welcome to your new dietary home! Phase 2 is a little more generous than Phase 1 in terms of carbohydrates, but it's still very much a low-carb approach. This phase is intended for people who feel their best on a low-carb diet but whose health and weight status don't require the degree of restriction of Phase 1. It's also where many people will be for the long term after following Phase 1 for some time and dramatically improving or perhaps even completely resolving the health issues they started with.

Phase 2 is a good place to start if you're already healthy and want to stay that way over the long term or if you're living with just one relatively minor health concern without complication from multiple others—for example, if you have gout or hypertension but no signs or symptoms of other problems. The Phase 2 carb allowance will likely be effective for improving your condition, but if you've experienced no improvement after several weeks or a few months, follow Phase 1 for a while. It's possible the more generous carb ceiling of Phase 2 is just a little too high for you to get the metabolic effects your body needs to heal.

> If you were **previously** consuming a **large amount of carbohydrate** and it led you to **metabolic disease** and **excess body fat**, that doesn't mean you can never consume any carbohydrates. It **means** you have to **learn how to use them** without harming yourself. **Phase 2** is intended to **help you** do this.

Notice I said *follow* Phase 1 for a while. I didn't say "go down to" Phase 1. Following Phase 1 isn't a demotion or a punishment. Don't be discouraged if you find yourself there. In fact, this is a good thing! You've identified your carb threshold at the current point in time. In the future, you might be able to return to Phase 2 without regaining weight or triggering a recurrence of your health issues. Even if you do have a recurrence, there's still no reason to be angry or disappointed with yourself. You may feel relieved instead. You've discovered for sure that your body does best with the ultra-low-carb intake of Phase 1. Armed with that knowledge, you can stay with Phase 1 and be successful for life.

Phase 2 is a good strategy for family members who are living with some of the issues in the table in Chapter 6 but who would balk at the mere thought of going as low as 20 grams of carbs per day. They might experience substantial improvement in their health following the slightly higher-carb plan outlined for Phase 2, and they might be perfectly satisfied with this, even if they would benefit even more from Phase 1.

As I've mentioned previously, everyone's carbohydrate tolerance differs. Some people have a large, rapid, and long-lived insulin response to a relatively small amount of carbohydrate, whereas others can eat a bit more carbs and still be in fat-burning mode most of the time because carbs induce a much smaller insulin response in them. People with even higher carbohydrate tolerances—the people blessed with a ninja-like metabolism—can thrive while consuming even more carbs. ADAPT Your Life Phase 3 is for them. If you're somewhere in between, Phase 2 is for you.

If Phase 2 seems a bit nebulous, like a loosely defined gray area somewhere in between Phase 1 and Phase 3, that's exactly what it is. Other than the situations I've described, most people following Phase 2 will be people who started with Phase 1 and stayed there long enough to lose large amounts of weight or to achieve substantial improvements, or possibly even complete remissions, of the health issues that originally plagued them. Having experienced these beneficial changes, they're ready to experiment with increasing their carbohydrate intake to see if their diet can be a little more liberal while they maintain the great success they had with Phase 1. I'll walk you through how to do this at the end of this chapter. First, let's look at the Phase 2 food list.

ADAPT Your Life Diet Phase 2 Food List

This list is designed to keep your total carbohydrate intake to 50 grams or fewer per day. See Appendix C for a handy cheat sheet of the Phase 2 food list that you can photocopy to put on your fridge or keep in your purse, briefcase, or car. (Take a picture of it with your phone, too, so you'll always have it handy.)

Phase 2 includes everything from Phase 1 (see pages 73 to 76) *plus* you can add the following:

- **Increase your portion sizes of the Phase 1 salad greens and nonstarchy vegetables, if desired:** Up to 4 cups of salad greens plus 2 cups of nonstarchy vegetables per day (or 1 cup of nonstarchy vegetables and 1 cup of Phase 2 vegetables)

- **If you are at your goal weight, increase your portion sizes of high-fat items, if desired:**
  - **Oils, cream, butter:** Up to 3 tablespoons per day
  - **Mayonnaise:** Up to 2 tablespoons per day
  - **Avocado:** Up to 1 fruit per day
  - **Olives:** Up to 12 per day

You can have the following foods in limited amounts:

- **Phase 2 vegetables:** Up to 1 cup per day (measured uncooked), which is approximately the size of a fist. Includes everything from Phase 1 plus carrots, beets, rutabaga, turnips, and winter squash (acorn, butternut, hubbard, spaghetti).

- **Berries:** Up to ½ cup per day. Includes raspberries, strawberries, blackberries, blueberries, cranberries (unsweetened, fresh—not dried).

- **Stone fruits:** Up to 1 small-to-medium fruit per day. Includes apricots, nectarines, peaches, plums. (Fresh fruit only, not dried or canned, and no juice or nectar.)

- **Nuts and seeds:** Up to 2 ounces per day. All nuts and seeds are permitted, but go easier on cashews, peanuts, and pistachios because they're higher in carbs. Nuts and seeds are preferable to nut and seed butters, which are very common trigger foods and are easy to get out of control with. It's best to avoid nut and seed butters unless you're confident you won't overdo them.

- **Dairy:** Includes everything from Phase 1 plus the following:
  - **Yogurt:** Up to 1 cup per day. Choose plain, unsweetened yogurt or sugar-free flavored yogurt. Both regular and Greek-style yogurt are permitted as long as they contain no added sugar. Add cinnamon, artificial sweetener, or a zero-carb fruit-flavored syrup for flavor if desired.

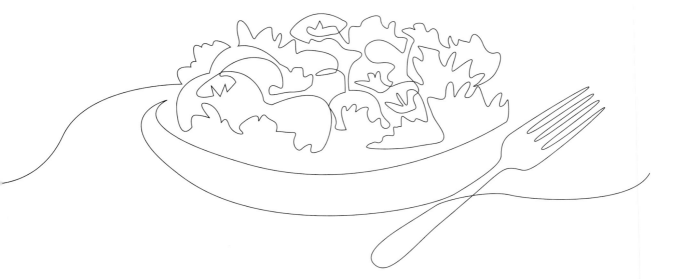

- **Cottage cheese:** Up to 1 cup per day. Choose plain, with no fruit or sugar added. Read the labels; some brands are higher in carbs than others. Most are 3 to 5 grams per ½ cup. (The same flavor suggestions for yogurt apply to cottage cheese.)
- **Ricotta cheese:** Up to ½ cup per day.

- **Low-carb grain products:** If you would like to add low-carb crispbreads, crackers, wraps, flatbreads, and the like to your diet, you may do so on Phase 2, but always read labels when purchasing these items and be vigilant about the *total carbohydrate*. Many of these products are marketed as "low-carb" or "keto," but because the ADAPT Your Life Diet counts total carbs without subtracting fiber, only some products will be suitable for you on Phase 2, and in limited quantities.

To ensure you don't exceed 50 grams of carbs per day, it's best to continue avoiding all beans, grains, and fruits apart from those I've specified. As always, read labels to make sure that your total carbohydrate intake for the day is 50 grams or fewer. As was true for Phase 1, these foods are what you *may* consume, not what you *must* consume while on Phase 2. You can mix and match the permitted foods to build a diet you enjoy. The most important thing is to stay under 50 grams of total carbs per day, so this might mean that you can't consume berries *and* stone fruit *and* yogurt *and* cottage cheese *and* nuts *and* low-carb grain products every day, but you can choose from among these to have more variety in your diet than you did on Phase 1, and a bit of variety from day to day if you choose.

Sample ADAPT Your Life Phase 2 Menus

Here's what a few days on Phase 2 might look like:

- **Breakfast:** Sausage patties with sautéed spinach; coffee or tea.
- **Lunch:** Cobb salad (romaine lettuce, hard-boiled egg, grilled chicken, diced tomato, blue cheese crumbles, bacon).
- **Dinner:** Lamb chops with roasted broccoli or butternut squash.
- **Dessert:** Sugar-free chocolate pudding made with avocado.
- **Snacks:** Carrot sticks and sliced cucumber with homemade sour cream and onion dip, ADAPT Keto Bar, Protein Bar, or Seed Bar (if you need to snack at all!).
- **Beverages:** Water, coffee, tea, sugar-free flavored beverages.

- **Breakfast:** Chaffles, which are "waffles" made from egg and shredded cheese; you can find recipes for chaffles, which can be savory or sweet, online. For sweet varieties, top with butter and sugar-free syrup, if desired. For savory, eat plain or add guacamole, salsa, or another topper.
- **Lunch:** Deli roast beef or turkey on a low-carb cracker with garlic and herb cream cheese; side of grilled zucchini or eggplant, if desired.
- **Dinner:** Grilled chicken over a Greek salad (lettuce, kalamata olives, feta cheese, cucumber, tomatoes, red onion; olive oil and red wine vinaigrette dressing); pair with pork rinds dipped in cauliflower hummus as an appetizer, if desired.
- **Dessert:** ½ cup of raspberries topped with unsweetened whipped cream, sour cream, or yogurt.
- **Snack:** Cottage cheese or yogurt topped with cinnamon and toasted sliced almonds or half a peach, sliced.
- **Beverages:** Water, coffee, tea, sugar-free flavored beverages.

- **Breakfast:** Leftover grilled chicken dipped in guacamole; coffee, tea.
- **Lunch:** Tuna or egg salad in lettuce wraps or a grain-based low-carb wrap.
- **Dinner:** Chinese takeout—chicken or shrimp with broccoli (steamed, no sauce; use soy sauce or hot mustard for flavor); side of steamed vegetables; augment with homemade cauliflower rice and garnish with sliced almonds or cashew halves, if desired.
- **Snacks:** Salami, 1 ounce of macadamia nuts, canned mackerel, small plum, ADAPT Keto Bar, Protein Bar, or Seed Bar.
- **Beverages:** Water, coffee, tea, sugar-free flavored beverages.

See Chapter 12 for additional Phase 2 meal and snack ideas.

Tips for Success on Phase 2 of the ADAPT Your Life Diet

Consume More of Your Carbohydrates Later in the Day

You may choose to have a very low-carb breakfast and lunch and consume a larger amount of vegetables with your evening meal or make dinner a large entrée salad. Eating very low-carb meals for most of the day can help you stay in ketosis until the evening. Even if you consume most of your carbs with your evening meal, the total amount permitted on Phase 2 is low enough that you will likely wake up in a deep fat-burning state again.

Use Caution with Fruit

Select fruits are permitted in limited quantities on Phase 2, but if you find that these small amounts of fruit trigger cravings for more, or trigger sugar cravings in general, consider staying fruit-free and increasing your carbs with larger portions or a broader variety of nonstarchy vegetables.

Know Yourself

If you're not able to control your portions of nuts and seeds, it's best to stay away from them. With common trigger foods, many people find it's easier to abstain completely than to consume the foods in moderation. (Isn't trying to eat certain things "in moderation" what gets so many people into metabolic trouble in the first place? If you can't be moderate, *don't consume these foods at all*.)

A Note for Postpartum Women

If you're postpartum and are trying to lose the weight you gained during pregnancy, the table in Chapter 6 pointed you to Phase 2. If your case is uncomplicated, meaning that you have no medical or health issues, and your only aim is to lose the "baby weight," Phase 2 is the right place for you. However, if you have health concerns aside from losing weight, you will be better served by starting with Phase 1. If you are currently breastfeeding, be aware that whichever phase of the ADAPT Your Life Diet you start with, you might need slightly more carbohydrate to support an adequate milk supply. Most women can breastfeed without incident when following Phase 1 or Phase 2, but some will find that a higher intake of starch works best for them. If this is the case for you, consume the amount of carbohydrate that best supports your milk supply and nourishes your baby for the duration of breastfeeding. After your baby is weaned onto solid foods, you can reduce your carb intake to a level that will be more effective for helping you lose body fat and improving other issues you may be living with.

Transitioning from Phase 1 to Phase 2 of the ADAPT Your Life Diet

I mentioned in Chapter 7 that some people who are successful in reaching their goal weight or resolving health issues by following Phase 1 may choose to remain on Phase 1 indefinitely, whereas others may prefer to transition to Phase 2 and partake of a higher amount and a wider variety of carbohydrates. I used the word "transition" deliberately because this process is just that: a transition. You don't *jump* to Phase 2; it's a gradual shift that allows you to systematically increase your carbs while maintaining all the beneficial changes you experienced on Phase 1. You will be tempted to go straight to 50 grams per day, but increasing your carbs slowly and systematically is the best way to identify your personal threshold without triggering weight regain or recurrence of health issues you were happy to be rid of on Phase 1.

Do not immediately increase from 20 grams to 50 grams of carbohydrate. You have been consuming a very low amount of carbohydrate for an extended period of time. To be able to identify your carbohydrate tolerance threshold, you will need to introduce Phase 2 foods slowly and methodically. Don't go from 20 grams of carbs a day to 50 grams overnight. The limit to stay under is 50 grams; that's not a target to aim for. Work your way up gradually. The way to do this is to increase your carb intake by 5 to 10 grams per week. Not per day; per *week*.

> " You will be **tempted** to **go straight** to 50 grams, but increasing your carbs **slowly** and **systematically** is the **best way** to identify your personal threshold and not trigger weight regain or recurrence of health issues you were happy to be rid of on **Phase 1**.

This means that if you were eating 20 grams of carbs per day on Phase 1, the first week you move to Phase 2, you'll consume 25 to 30 grams per day. The second or third week, you'll consume 30 to 35 grams per day, increasing the daily amount by 5 to 10 grams each week. It's up to you how quickly to proceed. You might choose to go very gradually and stay at 25 or 30 grams for two to four weeks, then increase to 35 or 40 grams for another few weeks, and so on. Whatever approach you choose, gradual is the name of the game. It's not a race. Going slowly will give you time to assess how you feel and to see whether your weight and blood sugar are staying in check as you increase your carbs.

A good way to start is to consume larger portions of the salad greens and nonstarchy vegetables you were already eating on Phase 1. After that, add 5- to 10-gram portions of new foods from Phase 2 each week. Here are some of the Phase 2 foods and the portion sizes that constitute 5 grams of carbs:

- **Nuts and seeds:** 1 ounce (cashews, peanuts, and pistachios are slightly higher in carbs; go easy)
- **Blueberries:** ¼ cup
- **Raspberries:** ⅓ cup
- **Strawberries:** 6 medium berries
- **Cottage cheese:** ½ cup
- **Yogurt (plain, unsweetened):** ½ cup
- **Carrots:** 1 medium-sized

Don't stress over getting this exactly right. Remember, the ADAPT Your Life Diet is designed to be simple and doesn't require weighing and measuring your food. If you're uncomfortable with eyeballing things, use measuring cups or a food scale for a few days until you feel more confident that you won't overdo the carbs. The main thing is to increase gradually and stick to the foods on the list. If you do that, you won't need to worry about every little fraction of a carb gram—what I call *carblets*.

Eating this way is not an exact science. You won't have the same appetite every day; you don't need to eat the same amount of food or number of carb grams every day. Stay within the framework, stick to the list, and don't worry about nailing the numbers 100 percent precisely.

> **Phase 2** is infinitely **customizable**, but keeping **total carbs low** is still the **most important aspect**. You'll be **eating more** carbs than on **Phase 1**, but you'll increase them in a **sensible, controlled way** that helps you **identify** your sweet spot.

Because your total carb intake is still somewhat limited, a smart way to go about the gradual increase for Phase 2 is to keep your breakfasts very low carb, which is easy to do because breakfast is often low in carbs anyway (eggs, bacon, sausage, cheese, etc.). Consider having more of your carbs with your lunch or dinner—an entrée salad with a protein source and more vegetables than you were eating on Phase 2, for example, or a fatty source of protein and a side dish of roasted beets or carrots for dinner. Alternatively, you can eat all your meals as if you're still on Phase 1 but add a small amount of berries with crème fraiche or peaches with cream for dessert.

ADAPT Your Life Phase 2 is infinitely customizable, but keeping total carbs low is still the most important aspect. You'll be eating more carbs than you were on Phase 1, but you'll increase them in a sensible, controlled way that helps you identify your sweet spot where your diet can be a little broader as you maintain the benefits you achieved with Phase 1.

To be clear, you don't *have* to move to Phase 2 at all. Some people are perfectly content with the food options on Phase 1 and have no desire to increase carbs. But many others prefer to broaden things. If you're in the second category, you will be able to do so while remaining free of the excess weight and the health issues Phase 1 helped you get rid of. Remember, with a limit of 50 total grams of carbohydrate per day, Phase 2 is still most definitely a low-carb diet. (Remember that 50 is a maximum, not a minimum. It's a limit to stay under rather than a target to aim for.) If chronically high blood sugar and insulin were driving your health problems in the past, it wasn't 50 grams of carbs per day that were responsible; it was probably more like 200 or 300 grams.

This being said, another approach after healing with Phase 1 is to follow Phase 1 most of the time but make occasional visits to Phase 2. If increasing your carbohydrate intake makes you nervous, be strategic about consuming more carbs. For example, your body will be better equipped to handle more carbs, metabolically speaking, on days when you do strenuous exercise. (You can consume the additional carbs at any time of day, but it's best to save them for after your workout.) You could also reserve higher-carb days for when you are traveling and might find it more difficult to stick to 20 grams of carbs or fewer. (The truth is, sticking to 20 grams while you're away from home is pretty simple—see Chapter 13 for tips—but it might ease your mind to know you have flexibility with a bit more carbs if your food options are limited on the road.)

You could also reserve higher-carb days for special occasions or when you're dining at a particular establishment where there's something very special or a family favorite on the menu or when you simply want to partake in more carbs than usual. As I explained for Phase 1, on Phase 2, your results might be equally good if you eat anything you want as long as your total carb intake for the day is 50 grams or fewer. The foods on the list are less likely to lead to cravings for more and more compared to other things that you could, technically, squeeze into a

50-gram limit, such as bread, pasta, cereal, ice cream, or cookies. What does this mean? It means you might be able to enjoy a piece of wedding cake, potato latkes at Hanukkah, pumpkin pie at Thanksgiving, or some chocolate eggs for Easter, but you are probably better served avoiding those most of the time. Occasional treats like these should be just that: occasional.

A Closer Look at Phase 2

Remember the sound modulator from Chapter 7? After following ADAPT Your Life Phase 1 for a while and having the diet dial turned up all the way, you're an old pro at keeping your carbs very low. Eating the foods that work best for you doesn't require as much dedicated thought as it did when you were new to the ADAPT Your Life Diet. Now it might be time to turn your attention to some of the other dials. Diet is still a major focus, though, and you don't want to take your eyes off its dial for so long that old habits creep back in, causing you to lose some of the ground you gained with Phase 1. You can remain vigilant about diet while also starting to look at other aspects of your overall health and well-being. It's like driving a car: You always keep your eyes on the road ahead of you, but you also need to be aware of the cars behind you and to your right and left, not to mention glancing now and then at your speedometer, fuel gauge, and engine temperature. Monitoring multiple things at once when you're behind the wheel is no problem for you, and it's no different with your health.

Phase 1 is a corrective diet. Once issues have been corrected, you don't need to stay in the corrective phase. If you break your leg, you wear a cast while the bone heals, but once the healing is done, you remove the cast. The cast helped you heal, but that doesn't mean you need to wear it for the rest of your life. It was a corrective measure, and once it's served its purpose, you no longer need it. For some people, Phase 1 is like the cast. You may have needed a very strict approach to tackle a severe situation, but when your situation is much improved, you might not need to be quite as strict.

If you've lost the weight you were looking to lose, and you're satisfied with how your health has improved, now is the time to think about other issues on your triage list. You have more energy now. Are you taking advantage of this and being more active? Exercise wasn't required for you to lose weight or to experience the other benefits of Phase 1, but it can be a powerful tool for overall physical and psychological well-being, not to mention that it gives you slightly more wiggle room for carbs.

Do you get sufficient sleep, or have you bought so much coffee in recent years that you've single-handedly put your favorite barista's kids through college? If you suspect that an inadequate amount or poor quality of sleep is standing in the way of feeling even better, consider the changes you would need to make to get better sleep.

Did ADAPT Your Life Phase 1 help restore your physical health, but your mental and emotional health are suffering from chronic stress? Now is the time to start looking for ways to reduce your stress load or find techniques that can help you cope better if reducing the total load is not possible. (Let's be realistic; sometimes it isn't possible.) If you juggle multiple jobs, care for a sick loved one, are a single parent, are going through a divorce, or are living with some other situation that may need a long time to resolve, it might be difficult to reduce the number of obligations and responsibilities you face. What *is* possible is finding ways to help you handle the stress better, even if only for a few minutes here and there throughout the day. You don't have to abandon your life and hop a flight to the nearest tropical island, although that would be nice if you can! It could be as simple as watching a funny video, listening to a favorite song on your phone, or engaging in positive self-talk when you need to. And don't forget the power of simply physically walking away from a situation for a moment to take some deep breaths.

When you started Phase 1, you had reasons why you wanted to feel better, and now you are feeling better. So, are you engaging with those reasons? Are you doing the things you wanted to do? Living the way you envisioned living on the other side of the weight, the fatigue, the aches and pains? Are there things in your life besides your diet that can make things even better? Phase 1 brought you this far. Phase 2 can help you go further.

Will I Ever Be at Phase 3?

If you started with Phase 1 due to long-standing obesity, metabolic syndrome, or multiple other issues stemming from insulin resistance, Phase 2 will probably be your permanent home. It's unlikely that you will be able to transition permanently to Phase 3, but you might be able to make occasional visits there, such as when you're on vacation to another country and want to experience the local cuisine or when there's another reasonable opportunity to temporarily—and I stress *temporarily*—consume more carbs than usual. (I would never tell you not to partake of a fresh croissant if you're in Paris for the first time or a scoop of gelato if you're touring Rome. Visiting the Caribbean? Allow yourself to have the black beans and plantains. Like I said earlier, these high-carb foods won't land you back in the thick of obesity or a metabolic illness as long as you have them only *occasionally*.)

Remember, the ADAPT Your Life Diet isn't a prison sentence. If eating a certain way led you to type 2 diabetes, obesity, metabolic syndrome, hypertension, pain and fatigue, or anything else that was reducing your quality of life, why would you want to go back there? If you've been hitting your thumb with a hammer and it hurts, the first order of business is to put the hammer down. The next order of business is never to pick it up again!

This comparison might be a little simplistic, though. Let me talk through this a little more clearly concerning dietary carbohydrate. Hammers are useful tools when used carefully, but they can be dangerous when handled carelessly. You don't need to avoid hammers altogether just because they can cause injury; use them correctly for their intended purpose, and there's no problem. If you were previously consuming a large amount of carbohydrate and you found yourself dealing with metabolic disease and excess body fat, that doesn't mean you can never consume any carbohydrates again. It means you have to learn how to use them without harming yourself. ADAPT Your Life Phase 2 is intended to help you do this—to enjoy carbohydrates in the form of select vegetables, fruits, dairy products, and nuts and seeds—but to keep the total amount within a level that doesn't trigger the pain and injury of the pasta, bread, and sugar hammers hitting you square in the face as they did in the past.

From Obesity, Sleep Apnea, IBS, and GERD to Healthy and Carb-Tolerant

"Restoring my metabolic health has made me able to handle a bit more starch just as well as it does my normal lower-carb, higher-fat days."

In January 2013, I was having lunch with my uncle, wife, and newly adopted daughter. We had just come from a morning at the zoo. My uncle, a math graduate from UC Berkeley, was one of the most brilliant people I've ever known. He was my science, literature, and thinking guide growing up. We read all the science heavyweights and great literature together. On this day, though, he could not remember having been at the zoo ten minutes prior.

My heart was breaking, again. It broke anew almost every day since he had been diagnosed with Alzheimer's. He was in his early seventies. His mother, my grandmother, died in her early sixties from type 2 diabetes after having her leg amputated. I was not doing well myself. I was forty-seven years old and had been morbidly obese for more

With an upper limit of 50 grams per day, Phase 2 is obviously still a very low-carb diet. You may be able to go higher than this amount, particularly if you're very physically active. If you have a history of metabolic illness or you know that too many carbs in your diet sets you up for cravings, insatiable hunger, or other issues that went away and stayed away on Phase 1 or Phase 2, you can experiment with the lower end of the carb spectrum on Phase 3—perhaps 75 to 80 grams per day or fewer, best limited to days when you exercise or are otherwise substantially active. It's unlikely, however, that you'll be able to consume the same amount of carbs as someone who has always been healthy, lean, and fit. Remember: It felt so good when you put that hammer down and your thumb healed. Don't start hitting it again! If you've been unwell for a significant length of time, Phase 2 isn't limiting; it's liberating.

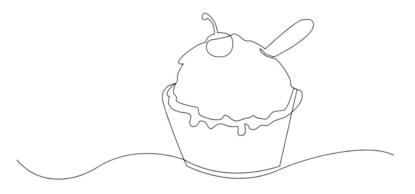

than twenty years. I spent ten years over 350 pounds (159 kg) and another decade between 260 and 300 (118 to 136 kg). (I am 5'9" [175 cm].) I had sleep apnea, severe allergies, GERD, IBS, daily gut pain, and all five markers of metabolic syndrome. My wife was also morbidly obese. That day after the zoo, I saw myself passing before my uncle, leaving my wife and two-year-old daughter alone.

I didn't take immediate action, but my health state weighed on me. In addition to the physical symptoms I've mentioned, I also had brain fog, depression, and anxiety, and I was constantly tired, hungry, and irritable. By May 2013 (four months after the zoo visit), I'd had enough of being sick and tired. I dedicated myself to solving things. I started my college career in chemical engineering, was briefly in molecular biology, then received a BA and MS in geography. I also had three years of a PhD program in geography. I had both a hard science background and a background in cultural ecology, which focuses on how traditional cultures use their resources for optimal health. It proved to be a good combination, and evenings and weekends were dedicated to researching my conditions.

I started by throwing out everything I'd heard about nutrition. Every food and claim had to make its case to me. I asked myself some important questions. I had noticed I was always hungry, and calories didn't seem to matter. I had fast-food meals two or three times a week. I always had unsweetened iced tea but with fries and a big burger with the works. Often these meals were 1,500 calories or more by themselves. But I was hungry soon after. Why? And why was my body fat? Wasn't fat there to be used? I also wondered if there was a connection between my grandmother's type 2 diabetes and my uncle's Alzheimer's. Was it a form of diabetes?

These questions led me to the concepts of metabolic syndrome, hyperinsulinemia, and insulin resistance as the root causes of all my various health conditions and psychological issues. There was emerging evidence on the internet of people having success reversing metabolic syndrome by greatly reducing and eliminating sugar, refined carbohydrates, certain oils, and grains. This was the Primal/Paleo movement combined with low-carb. It made so much sense to me because the diet was essentially the same one our ancestors and modern hunter-gatherers used. It perfectly aligned with my cultural ecology background. If it worked for them, why not for me?

So, I gave up all bread and pasta, candy, and potato chips right away. It worked amazingly well. Although I lost only two pounds of weight the first month, I had more physical and mental energy than I could ever remember. I was also less hungry than ever. After about three months, the weight loss really ramped up. I weighed 290 (131 kg) in May 2013; by the holidays, I was in the 230s (about 104 kg) and feeling incredible!

Shortly before the holidays, I experimented with white rice and beans at a Mexican restaurant. I hadn't had starchy vegetables, white rice, or any beans for months. I expected my hunger to increase, to experience hypoglycemia, and generally to feel sluggish and depressed. It didn't happen. The meal, which also included lots of meat and veggies but no corn chips and tortillas, left me feeling great and satisfied. It was an early lunch, and I was so full I didn't eat dinner. By this time, skipping breakfast was my new normal. I'd have two meals a day, or sometimes just one meal. I was doing time-restricted eating naturally because by eating real food and lowering my insulin levels, I was running on my own body fat, so I wasn't hungry that often.

But why did I do so well with white rice and beans? Within days of eating those carbs, I experienced noticeable fat loss and felt less hunger than normal. Why? It turns *out that white rice and beans are whole foods. Except for removing the bran from the rice, they're whole and intact—no refining, no being made into flour, bread, or chips. They're also not sugar. They're mostly glucose with very little fructose, which gives these foods a different effect on blood sugar and insulin. By the time I had experimented with these foods, I had lost a significant amount of weight and was more insulin sensitive. Being low-carb most of the time meant that my body had a little more room for starch once in a while, so I handled these whole-food carbs just fine.*

I started incorporating higher-carb meals (from whole-food, nonsugar carbs) about once every one to two weeks for the rest of my fat loss journey, from 230 pounds (104 kg) down to 170 (77 kg). I reached that weight in the fall of 2014, about eighteen months after I started. I also discovered longer intermittent fasting and extended fasting. This works very well for me, although it is not required for success with this way of eating. I have maintained my weight and gotten stronger and healthier by keeping the base of my diet low-carb whole foods, no grains, very low sugar, and appropriate amounts of fasting. This approach allows me to maintain all the benefits of a very low-carb diet while also periodically having all kinds of whole-food carbs, like potatoes and sweet potatoes.

I do not follow a "keto diet" by daily carb grams. However, because I eat mostly low-carb whole foods and do intermittent fasting, I am always fat-adapted and burning either my body fat or fat from my food for fuel. I spend part of each day in ketosis via a base of a low-carb diet, no snacking, and exercise. I find this a wonderful way to live and have exceptional health. I eat a variety of starches now but still avoid grains, except for white rice on rare occasions. My higher-carb days are typically around 120 to 150 grams of carbs, 200 grams very occasionally. These are no problem at all for me. Restoring my metabolic health has made me able to handle a bit more starch just as well as it does my normal lower-carb, higher-fat days.

I didn't do this alone. My wife has lost 70 pounds (32 kg) and also reversed many health conditions with this same way of living. Our daughter is a "real food kid," very low sugar, and she's thriving. This journey has also changed my career. I have the wonderful good fortune to now be a wellness coach and assistant researcher for medical professionals who are friendly to low-carb, keto, and intermittent fasting. I take incredible pleasure in helping my clients become fat-burning beasts for life!

—Larry D., Austin, TX

CHAPTER 9

ADAPT YOUR LIFE DIET PHASE 3

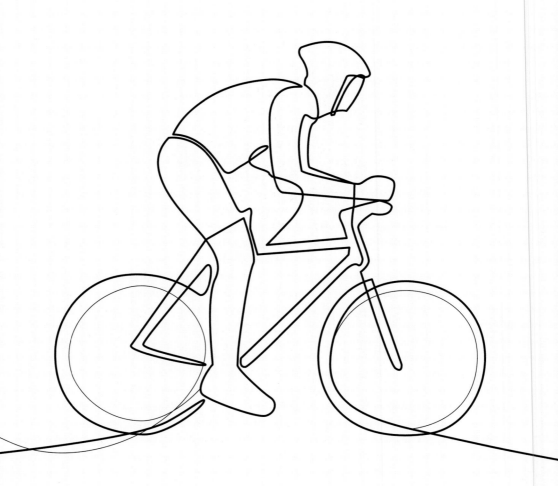

You'll start with Phase 3 of the ADAPT Your Life Diet if you're healthy and fit and simply want to follow a nutritious and sustainable way of eating to maintain your good health over the long term. This phase is the most generous phase in terms of carbohydrates—up to 150 total grams per day. In addition to the foods permitted on Phases 1 and 2, Phase 3 allows you to incorporate beans, grains, starchy vegetables, and more fruit if you choose to, but refined sugars are still off-limits. Remember, sugar provides you with nothing beneficial. As I explained in Part 1, it actually takes *away* from your body's nutrient status.

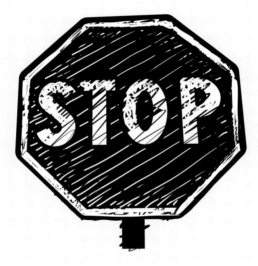

Fig 9.1: Wait! You didn't just jump right here to Phase 3, did you? Be sure to read about Phases 1 and 2 in Chapters 7 and 8 before moving on.

Don't be fooled into thinking that being lean and active is guaranteed protection against metabolic disease. It's not unusual for professional athletes to develop type 2 diabetes and other issues related to chronically high insulin or blood sugar. You can't out-exercise a bad diet. Your hormones and your blood sugar know exactly what you're eating, and you can't fool them with running, biking, or swimming. Many athletes can eat anything and everything they want and remain lean and healthy when they're young, but their eating habits catch up with them when they're older. It's not uncommon to see a former pro athlete who's packed on the pounds after they retire from their sport because they continue eating like someone who exercises for a living long after their career has come to a close.

You might have even seen some of them become spokespeople for commercial weight-loss programs, starring in infomercials that try to sell you shakes and pills. Don't become one of these people. Understand ADAPT Your Life Phase 1 and Phase 2, master Phase 3, and you'll be able to stay metabolically healthy no matter what your physical activity level is like.

Most people, no matter how lean and active they are, will not be in a ketogenic state at the higher end of the Phase 3 carb spectrum. You might occasionally enter ketosis if you have a day here and there where you consume fewer carbs than usual. You also might wake up in a ketogenic state because your insulin level will be low first thing in the morning, and you will have used up some of your liver glycogen stores during the night. (In fact, for some people, "morning breath" is probably actually keto breath!) If you mostly stay at the higher-carb end, though, you probably won't be in ketosis most of the time. But that's fine—remember, if you're at Phase 3, you don't *need* the power of ketosis.

> Compared to what most people in modern industrialized societies are eating, **Phase 3** is *relatively* **low in carbohydrate**, but compared to Phases 1 and 2, there's a **lot of flexibility** for carb intake. Ketogenic and very low-carb diets are **not the only ways** to be lean and healthy.

Phase 3 is different from Phases 1 and 2 because it is not designed to be ketogenic or very low carb. Compared to what most people in modern industrialized societies are eating, Phase 3 is *relatively* low in carbohydrate, but compared to Phases 1 and 2, there's a lot of flexibility for carb intake. It's obvious that ketogenic and very low-carb diets are not the only ways to be lean and healthy. As I noted earlier, people all over the world remain lean, healthy, and free of chronic metabolic illness without following ketogenic diets. (What would the traditional Japanese diet be without rice, or Central American cuisine without corn?) The reason some people can consume liberal amounts of carbohydrates with no adverse effects is that their physiology may naturally be better suited to do so.

But there's an even more important reason—one that's relevant to you if the table in Chapter 6 led you to Phase 3 but which is also relevant to people starting at Phase 1 or Phase 2: If you've always been healthy, then you don't need to *get* healthy. If you've never been sick, you don't need to *reverse* illness. If you've never been overweight, and you don't have a sweet tooth, you don't know what brain fog is, your energy level is high most of the time, you've had clear skin all your life except for a blip on the hormonal radar during puberty, and a doctor has never expressed concern about any of your blood tests, then you have good metabolic flexibility, and you don't need ketosis to feel your best.

> "If you've **always been** healthy, then you **don't need** to *get* healthy. If you've **never been** sick, you **don't need** to *reverse* illness. If you have good metabolic flexibility, **you don't need ketosis** to feel your best.

What's metabolic flexibility? It's the ability to move seamlessly from being fueled by carbs to being fueled by fat and back again. You feel equally good whether your diet is a bit higher in carbs on some days or a bit lower. You efficiently convert carbs *and* fat into energy, and your body doesn't have a preference for one over the other.

If you're starting with Phase 3, your body responds better to carbohydrates than does that of someone who checked several boxes in the table in Chapter 6. When you eat carbs, your blood sugar and insulin rise less than theirs do, and the levels come back down to normal more quickly for you as well. You have a higher carb tolerance, which is why you can skip Phases 1 and 2 and slide right into Phase 3. (However, as I mentioned in Chapter 7, you might choose to start with Phase 1 anyway to see whether there are any specific benefits you experience while in ketosis.)

Remember, Phase 1 is a corrective diet. You don't need to correct a problem you don't have. In Chapter 8, I used the example of a broken leg. You'd wear a cast to help a broken leg heal, but you wouldn't put a cast on a healthy leg as a protective measure to prevent it from breaking. The very strict ketogenic approach of Phase 1 is what will correct many serious health issues most quickly and effectively. If you don't have a serious health issue, you don't need the strictest approach.

Let's revisit the sound modulator. If you're in Phase 3, your diet dial doesn't need to be turned up all the way. Diet is not unimportant, but on Phase 3, you have the flexibility to be more liberal with your diet, and you can give more attention to other aspects of overall health and well-being.

The ADAPT Your Life Diet Phase 3 Food List

This list is designed to keep your total carbohydrate intake to 150 grams or fewer per day on most days. See Appendix C for a handy cheat sheet of the Phase 3 food list that you can photocopy to put on your fridge or keep in your purse, briefcase, or car or take a photo to keep on your phone.

Phase 3 includes everything from Phase 1 and Phase 2 (see pages 73 to 76 and 127 to 129) *plus* you can incorporate the following:

- **You can have unlimited salad greens and nonstarchy vegetables.**
- **If you are at your goal weight, increase your portion sizes of high-fat items, if desired:**
  - **Oils, cream, butter:** Up to 4 tablespoons per day
  - **Mayonnaise:** Up to 3 tablespoons per day
  - **Avocado:** 1 whole fruit per day
- **Fruits: Add citrus (grapefruit, tangerine, oranges); melon (all varieties); tropical fruits (mango, papaya, pineapple, kiwi).** Note that if you choose to include fruit in your diet, fresh, whole fruit is best, and it's still best to avoid fruit juice. Even if you have a high carbohydrate tolerance, juice is liquid sugar and is best avoided. Dried fruit is okay if it contains no added sugar, but be mindful of the total carbs. Dried fruits are concentrated sources of natural sugar, and the carbs will add up more quickly than for fresh fruit. (These might be best reserved to take along on a long training run or cycling ride since they're lightweight and will give you a quick energy boost.)
- **Starchy roots and tubers:** Potatoes, sweet potatoes, yams, parsnips, and all other starchy root vegetables.
- **Beans, legumes, and pulses:** All varieties (black beans, kidney, navy, turtle, lima, garbanzos, lentils, and all other beans and pulses).
- **Grains:** Corn, wheat, rice, oats, millet, amaranth, spelt, and barley.

So, What Do I Eat?

As you can see, except for sugar, no foods are off-limits on Phase 3. However, Phase 3 isn't a license to eat unlimited starches and fruits. Remember, you can't fool your bloodstream—no matter how much exercise you do. (See Glen F.'s story at the end of this chapter.) Even on Phase 3, it's not a great idea to have bottomless breadsticks as an appetizer before your pasta dinner and follow it up with an ice cream sundae. You still have a limited carbohydrate allowance; spend it wisely. As was true for the 50-gram carb limit for Phase 2, the 150-gram daily cutoff for

Phase 3 is a limit to stay *under*, not a target to aim for. Depending on your activity level and overall health, you might feel best staying at the lower end of Phase 3, maybe around 75 grams per day. Others might feel their best at closer to 150 grams.

> "Except for sugar, **no foods** are **off-limits** on **Phase 3**. However, Phase 3 **isn't a license** to eat unlimited starches and fruits. Remember, **you can't fool** your **bloodstream**—no matter how much exercise you do. Even professional athletes **aren't immune** to cardiometabolic **diseases** driven by **high blood sugar** or **insulin**.

So what does the limit look like in terms of the carbs in your diet? For 30 grams of carbs, you can have 1 cup of grapes or *1½ pounds* (0.7 kg) of cauliflower. For about 27 grams of carbs, you can have one medium-sized banana, 1 cup of chopped carrots, ½ cup of sliced strawberries, 1 cup of cubed eggplant, *and* 1 cup of chopped zucchini. Not that I recommend eating those things together! I'm just making the point that the *type* of carbohydrate foods you choose will determine the *amount* of them that you can eat while staying within your personal carb tolerance. Imagine the amount of lower-carb vegetables and fruits you could eat for the 46 grams of carbs in 1 cup of cooked brown rice, or the nearly 40 grams in 1 cup of cooked quinoa. If you prefer to consume a smaller quantity of more carb-dense foods, you have the flexibility to do that with Phase 3. However, if you tend to have a big appetite and would rather eat a larger volume of food, stick with foods that are a little lower in carbs so you can consume more of them in total. As you can see, Phase 3 provides the most variety and the most freedom to customize things.

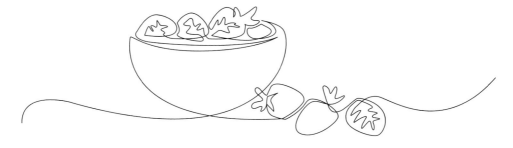

Sample ADAPT Your Life Phase 3 Menus

Here's what a few days on Phase 3 might look like:

- **Breakfast:** Veggie and cheese omelet; small bowl of fruit salad, if desired; coffee or tea
- **Lunch:** Couscous or whole-grain salad with a protein source (chicken, fish)
- **Dinner:** Chicken and steak fajitas (with onions, red and green peppers), with or without tortillas; side of rice or cauliflower rice, sour cream
- **Snacks:** Mixed nuts; melon wedges, ADAPT Keto Bar, Protein Bar, or Seed Bar
- **Beverages:** Water, coffee, tea, sugar-free flavored beverages

- **Breakfast:** Western omelet (eggs, diced onion, ham, green pepper), slice of whole wheat toast or serving of potato home fries; coffee or tea
- **Lunch:** Indian takeout—chicken or lamb over lentils or rice; small piece of naan bread, if desired
- **Dinner:** Beef or turkey meatballs with tomato sauce over zucchini noodles or wheat spaghetti
- **Dessert:** A few squares of dark chocolate
- **Snack:** Hard-boiled eggs, ADAPT Keto Bar, Protein Bar, or Seed Bar
- **Beverages:** Water, coffee, tea, sugar-free flavored beverages

- **Breakfast:** Oatmeal or corn grits with butter, cream, or other fat source; eggs, sausage, or other protein; coffee, tea
- **Lunch:** Chicken salad sandwich or lettuce wrap
- **Dinner:** Grilled steak with sautéed mushrooms and a baked potato or mashed cauliflower
- **Snacks:** Canned sardines, hummus with vegetables or pita chips, ADAPT Keto Bar, Protein Bar, or Seed Bar
- **Beverages:** Water, coffee, tea, sugar-free flavored beverages

See Chapter 12 for additional Phase 3 meal and snack ideas.

Phase 3 Flexibility

Earlier, I said Phase 3 is designed to keep your carb intake to no more than 150 grams on most days. Some days you might choose to go a little higher. If you're very active or athletic, you can consume more than this on training days or days you're competing. You can experiment with consuming more than 150 grams on other days, too, but if you find you feel better physically, mentally, or cognitively at a lower carb intake, save the extra carbs for days when your body has a higher demand for them.

You *can* perform at your athletic best while following a very low-carb or ketogenic diet. More and more professional athletes are doing this, and some are achieving personal bests. They run the gamut from ultra-distance runners to cyclists, from weightlifters to MMA fighters. You might find you can perform your best at a very low carb intake, but don't worry if this doesn't describe you. Some people find they need slightly more carbs in their diet to hit their highest gear and maintain their best endurance, strength, or power output, so don't be afraid to consume more carbs if you need to. Remember, if you're already lean and very active, and particularly if you're young, your metabolic situation is very different from that of someone starting with Phase 1 owing to obesity or a serious medical condition. Not only do you have the tolerance for more carbohydrate, but depending on your training schedule, you might feel and perform *better* with more carbs.

An alternative to consuming more carbs daily is to incorporate some variation of "carb cycling" into your life. There are many different ways to implement carb cycling, but generally speaking, carb cycling calls for staying very low-carb most of the time and including a higher-carb day once a week or a few times a month. Some athletes find this approach allows them to reap the benefits of being in a fat-burning or ketogenic state most of the time while also performing at the top of their game.

> **150 grams** of carbs is a **limit** to **stay under**, not a **target to aim for**. You could choose to keep your carbs near the **low end of the Phase 3** spectrum most days and opt to have **more carbs on hard training days** or during recovery from an endurance event.

If you're reading this and your current situation points you to Phase 1 and just 20 grams of carbs per day, understand that not everyone has the kind of metabolic flexibility that will allow them to thrive on Phase 3. People who are lean and very physically active can safely handle more carbohydrates than those with metabolic illnesses. Punctuating a mostly low-carb approach with some higher-carb days on a regular basis can work for people in the former group because their muscles are hungry for the carbs, and they'll go right back to fat-burning a short time after the carb-up. On the other hand, if you have obesity or a health issue driven by high blood sugar or insulin, it could take several days for your body to get back to maximal fat-burning. This might be all right if overdoing your carbs is a rare—very rare—occurrence, but the more often you do this, the longer it will take you to get the results you want—if you get them at all.

Navigate Sensibly

Phase 3 obviously has the most generous allowance for carbohydrates. Depending on your activity level, weight, and health status at any given time, you might be at the high end of the range, or you might opt to stick to the lower end. If you're not sure which is best for you, work with your doctor and have bloodwork done regularly, which will allow you to monitor how you're doing, metabolically speaking. Hemoglobin A1c or triglycerides that start trending upward or body fat percentage that noticeably increases is a sign that your carb intake has been a little higher than it should be. If you have bloodwork done twice a year, you can correct things long before they have a chance to get out of hand.

I'm Healthy and Active. Can't I Just Eat Whatever I Want?

Maybe you can eat whatever you want, but you're reading this book because health is a priority for you, and perhaps optimizing your physical performance is also a priority. With this in mind, things are more complicated than just managing your carbohydrate intake. You could get 150 grams of carbs from cupcakes, beer, macaroni and cheese, and potato chips, but you wouldn't expect optimal health, athletic performance, or cognitive function from that. ADAPT Your Life Phase 3 is where you might shift focus from the quantity of carbs you consume to the quality of your overall diet.

Because you are unencumbered by excess body fat or major health problems, you might be better able to tell if particular foods work well for you. For example, endurance athletes are often plagued with digestive complaints or gastrointestinal discomfort in general, and during events in particular. Certain foods may aggravate these issues for you more than others. I normally recommend against tracking or recording food—remember, I'm trying to keep this as simple as possible—but if you're at a level where every bit of competitive edge matters, it might be a worthwhile endeavor for you to record what you eat and how it affects you physically and psychologically, and how your athletics or mental focus is altered. Things to note are your energy level, any digestive distress (acid reflux, bloating, belching, loose stools), mental sharpness, mood, and parameters related to your physical performance.

Transitioning from Phase 2 to Phase 3

It's uncommon for people transitioning from ADAPT Your Life Phase 2 to thrive on the higher end of the Phase 3 carb limit. Unless you are especially active and you've built a significant amount of muscle mass, you will likely do best staying toward the lower end, perhaps 75 to 100 grams per day or fewer. And even that might be best for occasional days here and there rather than being your daily pattern. The way to transition from Phase 2 to Phase 3 is the same as for going from Phase 1 to Phase 2: Don't increase your carb intake to 100 or 150 grams right away. If you're satisfied with your weight and you're healthy and active, then as you go from Phase 2 to Phase 3, you don't need to be quite as careful as someone who is transitioning from Phase 1 to Phase 2. Try increasing your carbs by 10 to 20 total grams per week.

I recommend starting by introducing larger quantities of salad greens and nonstarchy vegetables, which, as you saw in the food list, are unlimited on Phase 3. The reason they're unlimited is that when you're already healthy and lean, it's hard to consume so much broccoli, spinach, cucumbers, or mushrooms that their carbohydrates would negatively impact your metabolic health. After you've done this for a few weeks, a good next step is to incorporate some of the foods that are new for Phase 3, like starchy tubers (potatoes, yams), beans, or fruits that were not part of Phase 2. It's best to incorporate grains last.

Individual sensitivity in how different foods affect blood sugar and insulin varies a lot among people. Generally speaking, though, grain-based foods (cereal, granola, pasta, bread, crackers) tend to affect blood sugar and insulin more than the other carbohydrate sources on Phase 3. Plus, unless you're making homemade bread from scratch, a cooked wheatberry salad, or rice pilaf or couscous, it's almost impossible to find grain-based foods that don't have added sugar. As I've said, even when these products' packages are emblazoned with "Whole Grains!" and other marketing gimmicks, they typically contain sugar—often a lot of it. (Look at the labels on cereal boxes, especially cereals that boast of being high in fiber and made from whole grains. You'll be shocked at how much sugar they pack, and it's even more stunning when you see the serving sizes—usually only *1 cup*, or sometimes even less!—and most of us would be tempted to eat a lot more than that. High-fiber whole-grain bran muffins are even worse.)

When incorporating more carbs, make them the side dish rather than the main event. For example, have a small amount of pasta as an accompaniment to a meat dish; a big bowl of pasta shouldn't be the star of the meal. For breakfast, have a wedge of melon or a handful of berries as a sweet addition to your main meal of sausage and eggs rather than making a meal of cereal and toast.

> You **don't need** to consume the same amount of carbs or the same amount of food every day. Some days you'll find yourself very hungry, and you'll feel less so on others. **Your body isn't a machine**, so **don't expect** to consume the same number of calories *or carbs* every day.

I also recommend consuming more of your carbs later in the day, particularly on days you exercise or train hard. Staying low to very low carb for most of the day keeps your metabolism running primarily on fat and gives your liver and muscles time to use their stored carbohydrate (glycogen). When your glycogen stores are reduced, carbs will have somewhere to go when you consume them later in the day—your body is primed to use them to replenish this glycogen rather than to store them as fat or to keep all that glucose in your bloodstream for an extended amount of time. This strategy—consuming carbs in the evening, particularly if you've done a strenuous workout earlier in the day—is sometimes referred to as *carb backloading*.

These are just suggestions, though. You can increase your carbs and reintroduce higher-carb foods any way you like. The main thing, just as with ADAPT Your Life Phases 1 and 2, is to be aware of your total carbohydrate intake. And keep in mind that you don't need to consume the same amount of carbs or the same amount of food every day. Some days you'll find yourself very hungry, and you'll feel less so on others. Your body isn't a machine, so don't expect to consume the same number of calories *or carbs* every day.

When increasing your carb intake on Phase 3, be prepared for a slight increase in your scale weight. You're not gaining body fat; the extra weight comes from your body holding onto water, which is to be expected when you regularly eat more carbs. I previously mentioned that very low-carb diets have a natural diuretic effect, meaning that they cause your body to let go of water. When you increase your carb intake, especially if you're at the higher end of Phase 3, it's just the process happening in reverse: with more carbs in your diet, your body holds on to a bit more water.

If you're hesitant about increasing your carbohydrate intake toward the higher amounts on Phase 3, there are a couple of ways to approach things. First, you don't *have to* go as high as 150 grams. You could choose to stay at the lower end, perhaps 50 to 80 grams per day, all the time. You also could stay with this amount (or less) on days you're more sedentary and eat more carbs on hard training days. Beyond this, you can use a blood glucose meter if you'd like to see how the new foods you're introducing are affecting you. But the ADAPT Your Life Diet is designed for this to be unnecessary. Your body is the best meter out there. It'll tell you how you feel. You'll know whether issues that were resolved on Phase 1 or Phase 2 are creeping back after some time on Phase 3. If you'd like to be a little more methodical about monitoring but prefer to keep things low-tech, consider keeping a log to record what you eat, how much you eat, and how you feel physically, cognitively, mentally, and emotionally. A food journal can help you discover whether your body responds to certain foods better than others or if there's a sweet spot in terms of the quantity of higher-carb foods that works best for you.

Beyond Carbs

In talking about the sound modulator analogy earlier, I said that on Phase 3, your nutrition dial doesn't have to be turned up as much as for people following Phases 1 or 2. The reason is that if you start at a point where you're already healthy, active, and lean, then your health and your weight are not negatively affected by what you're eating, and you don't need as radical a change in your diet as someone who is in a severe health crisis. In a way, though, because you're already healthy and might be looking to take things to the maximum level, be it in athletic performance, cognitive function, work productivity, or some other aspect of your life, your nutrition is even *more* important.

If you were a professional race car driver, you would be a lot more selective about things like the tires on your car and the fuel you use compared to someone who uses their car for occasional trips to the store. You wouldn't put just any brand of gasoline in the tank, and you wouldn't have your crew buy the cheapest set of tires available. You'd want precision. The very best.

When it comes to food, this is where there might be a role for choosing certain foods over others. In the more than two decades I've been using the low-carb, ketogenic approach with my patients, I have not seen sticking to conventionally produced food to be an obstacle to anyone losing weight or resolving serious health problems. I want to be clear about this because you should not feel that shopping for food at your local supermarket will give you lesser results than procuring all your food from local farms or organic producers. However, the way foods are produced—animal foods, specifically (beef, pork, poultry, eggs, seafood, dairy, etc.)—does affect their nutrient content.

For example, the precise amounts of various types of fats in beef from cattle raised exclusively on grass or in pork raised on pasture with certain types of feed are different from those of animals raised in conventional feedlot settings. Slight differences exist in the nutrient content of dairy products from cows raised exclusively on grass, poultry raised outdoors or with specifically formulated feed rations, and seafood caught from the wild in its natural marine habitat compared to those that are conventionally farmed. With this in mind, if you have the means, you may want to consider buying more of your animal foods from local farms where animals are raised in more natural settings or to order from companies that will ship this type of food right to your door. Although the differences are slight, when you're looking for every possible angle by which to take things to the next level, this is one area you can explore if your budget allows.

Something else you might choose to think about on Phase 3 is the nature of your food. Athletes—especially endurance athletes—tend to get sidelined by things like colds and upper respiratory tract infections, sometimes multiple times a year. Your body might be better supported by whole, single-ingredient foods rather than items with long lists of ingredients you can't identify. What are "single-ingredient" foods? Foods that consist of *one thing*: Chicken. Lamb. Asparagus. Cabbage. Cantaloupe. Zucchini. Walnuts. Pineapple. Beef. Black beans.

To be honest, there isn't much science behind these suggestions, but when you want every potential advantage you can use to your benefit, you can experiment with making unprocessed foods the basis of your diet to see if you feel or perform better than when your diet includes greater amounts of highly refined and processed foods. Do you need a randomized controlled trial to tell you what's right for you, or does your body give you the best possible feedback?

Another area to evaluate on ADAPT Your Life Phase 3 is your use of sugar substitutes, which is a very controversial issue. For some people, being able to consume foods and beverages that contain artificial sweeteners and sugar alcohols is what allows them to stick to a lower-carb diet for the long haul, and I support this. (Remember to count the total carbs from products that contain sugar alcohols, though.) For most of my patients, artificial sweeteners (sucralose, saccharin, aspartame) don't interfere with fat loss or improving metabolic problems. Sugar alcohols are a bit murkier. Artificial sweeteners contribute a negligible amount of carbs and don't affect blood sugar for most people, but sugar alcohols can pack a surprising punch. There isn't a lot of room for these on Phase 1 or Phase 2 because the ADAPT Your Life Diet counts total carbs and doesn't subtract sugar alcohols, but Phase 3 is more flexible.

Several different kinds of sweetening agents fall under the category of sugar alcohols (such as xylitol, sorbitol, mannitol, maltitol, and erythritol). Some have a higher glycemic impact than others, and, of course, individual responses to these vary. Some people are barely affected by any of them, whereas others may experience a substantial rise in blood sugar. Beyond the unpredictable glycemic effects, sugar alcohols are notorious for causing bloating, gas, and loose stools when consumed in large quantities—and some people might experience these unpleasant issues even after consuming only a small amount. (Sugar-free chocolates sweetened with maltitol or mannitol typically come with a warning that they can have a laxative effect if overconsumed.) If you're looking to optimize every possible aspect of your digestion and physical performance, consider eliminating sugar alcohols from your diet or do some self-experimentation and see how different ones affect you. You might find that you're better off avoiding some but that others work just fine for you. (Erythritol typically has the least impact on blood sugar and digestion, but remember that individual responses vary.)

In following ADAPT Your Life Phase 3 and seeking to optimize all aspects of your health and performance, you might also consider the use of nutritional supplements more than someone following Phase 1 or Phase 2. If you're eating appropriate foods, supplementation is not necessary, but that doesn't mean certain compounds can't be beneficial. (A massage or an occasional glass of wine isn't necessary for a happy life, but they can certainly help those who enjoy them!)

A detailed discussion of different vitamins, minerals, and other compounds that have potential benefit for athletic performance or boosting focus is beyond the scope of this book, but here's some basic information to get you thinking about things that could potentially be useful for you:

- **Sodium:** Chapter 7 covered the importance of sodium. Many people on very low-carb diets need more sodium than they're accustomed to consuming. Even though Phase 3 is not an ultra-low-carb diet, you may be eating far less carbohydrate than you were in the past, so, relatively speaking, it's low carb for you. If you find yourself feeling sluggish, tired, and like you've lost your "oomph" when working out or training, increasing your sodium (salt) intake often resolves these issues quickly. (Headaches or feeling dizzy or lightheaded on a lower-carb diet are surefire signs that you need more sodium.)

- **Magnesium:** Magnesium is another critical mineral on lower-carb diets, particularly for those who routinely tax their muscles. Magnesium is a natural muscle relaxant, so supplemental magnesium can help if you experience muscle stiffness or cramps. Some people also find magnesium helps them fall asleep, so consider supplemental magnesium if you have trouble sleeping.

- **Protein powder:** If you're trying to build muscle mass and have trouble consuming enough whole food protein to support your efforts, protein powders may be helpful. Whey protein may be especially effective, but egg white protein is also available, and people with allergies to dairy or eggs can use pea, hemp, or rice proteins. (Really, though, if you want to increase your protein intake, I recommend just eating more meat or eggs!) Branched-chain amino acids (BCAAs) are favored in the bodybuilding community for use before or during workouts because your muscles can use them as quick fuel, but they don't have the adverse effects of that other quick fuel—glucose. BCAAs have also been shown to help reduce muscle soreness after exercise, which could aid in recovery.

- **L-glutamine:** Considering the negative impacts of endurance activity on the GI tract, some endurance athletes find that taking supplemental L-glutamine is beneficial. L-glutamine is an amino acid that fuels the cells that line the small intestine. Prolonged physiological stress may increase the body's need for glutamine, and although you can get enough from food, regularly engaging in high-intensity or long-duration exercise might mean that a little extra could be beneficial.

- **Ketones:** It's possible to supplement with ketones without being on a ketogenic diet. Supplemental ketones (called *exogenous* ketones, because they come from the outside rather than being made by your body) are now available, usually in the form of a powder that you add to water and consume as a beverage. Research is ongoing, but some athletes find that they experience a slight energy boost when taking exogenous ketones before a workout. I typically recommend against the use of these ketone products for people with obesity, diabetes, or other metabolic health problems, but if you're healthy and athletic, you may want to experiment with them to see whether they provide any type of physical advantage for you.

    Beyond physical performance, some people feel that exogenous ketones offer a cognitive boost, and a dose helps them with sharper thinking and better focus. Following a healthy diet and having steady blood sugar and insulin levels will accomplish this for most people without any extra supplementation, but again, you can experiment with exogenous ketones for this purpose if you want to.

- **MCT oil:** Another way people support cognitive function is by using oils consisting of medium-chain fatty acids (also called MCT oil), such as by putting it in their morning coffee or tea. Coconut oil contains a high percentage of these medium-chain fats, so coconut oil has a similar effect as straight MCT oil for some people. MCTs are digested differently than other fats, and they're more readily converted into ketones, so using these oils can raise ketone levels without the use of exogenous ketones. In fact, MCT oil and exogenous ketones can raise ketone levels even when you're on a high-carb diet, so if you experience a noticeable physical, mental, or cognitive benefit from ketones, you could try using these even on your higher-carb days. Ingesting large amounts of MCT oil or coconut oil can have a laxative effect, so start with a small amount and increase gradually if you want to experiment with these.

Please know that unlike the ADAPT Your Life Phase 1 dietary approach, which is supported by numerous scientific studies and has been successful for weight loss and disease remission in thousands of people from all walks of life, research into the use of MCT oil and exogenous ketones is in its early days. There is no guarantee that using them will be effective for you. That's not a reason not to try them, but you should consider them add-ons to the healthy diet and lifestyle you're already employing. Just like supplements, they are not intended to make up for bad habits; they are supplemental to the good things you're already doing. Experimenting with various nutritional supplements, ketones, and MCT oil are the last dials to adjust after you've addressed other aspects of your diet and lifestyle that are likely to have a bigger impact.

A Note About Overtraining

Feeling sluggish or tired, seeing a decline in your athletic performance, and perhaps even feeling anxious or depressed are not automatic indicators that you need more carbohydrates. If your carb intake has been at the low end of Phase 3 for a while and you've been training hard, it's possible you would feel significantly better if you increased your starch intake. Consume more carbohydrates, and you'll know within just a few days whether this was the issue. But if you increase your carbs significantly and you still feel like you're dragging physically and emotionally, consider that you might be experiencing overtraining syndrome.

Overtraining syndrome is sometimes informally referred to as *burnout* because that's exactly how it feels: like you're *burned out*. The following are some signs and symptoms to look out for:

 Fatigue

 Weight loss (or weight gain, less commonly)

 Difficulty focusing or concentrating

 Decline in performance

 Moodiness or personality changes

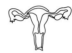 Frequent illness; decreased immune function

 Loss of enthusiasm for the sport or activity

 Anger or irritability

 Amenorrhea (loss of menstrual period in women of reproductive age)

 Insomnia or difficulty sleeping

 Prolonged recovery time

 Lower testosterone; loss of libido in men

 Loss of appetite

 Chronic injury; slow healing

Overtraining is exactly what it sounds like: training, exercising, or working out without giving your body adequate rest, recovery, and nutritional replenishment. Increasing your carbohydrate intake can help, but overtraining syndrome is your body's way of telling you that you need to back off on your training for a little while to give your body and mind a break. It doesn't mean you have to abandon your sport or activity altogether, but your body is giving you loud and clear signals that you're overdoing things—and probably have been for a while. Overtraining doesn't happen after just a few days or weeks. It's something that happens over a longer period when your body is depleted and no longer has the resources to be resilient in the face of overexertion.

With this in mind, letting up on your training frequency, volume, intensity, or all three will help, as will devoting time to physical and psychological rest and relaxation. It's beyond the scope of this book to delve any further into the subject of overtraining. Just be aware that if you're very athletic and routinely engage in either high-intensity or long-duration activities, and you begin to experience some of the issues I mentioned, your carbohydrate intake isn't the only factor to consider.

You've likely heard the phrase, "Train smarter, not harder." Sometimes training smarter means backing off a little. Pushing yourself to your limits every time you work out or train can backfire after months or years of keeping up that kind of relentless pace. Rather than making you stronger, fitter, and healthier, it can begin to erode your physical and mental health and end up doing the opposite of what you were trying to achieve. Most people in the modern industrialized world could probably benefit from putting more effort toward deliberate exercise and increasing physical activity in general, but if you're already working to your maximum and have been for a while, more isn't always better. You're not a failure if you need to cut back a bit, and your performance isn't automatically going to suffer. In fact, it might get *better* when you give your body the downtime it needs to recover.

Beyond Diet Altogether

When following ADAPT Your Life Phase 3, dials beyond diet and exercise become more important for supporting physical performance and recovery, cognition (focus, attention, memory, information processing), work productivity, and overall well-being. If you work hard, you need to rest hard, too. Respect that your body is not a machine. It needs a break from constant maximal effort, be it on a running trail, in the weight room, or in the boardroom. (Even machines, like your phone or your tablet, need to recharge, too!)

If you want your body to use the good food you give it to its maximal potential, you have to put that food into a system that's primed to take advantage of it. Back to the car metaphor: Why bother putting super-premium fuel into a car that has bald tires and hasn't had an oil change in two years? On Phase 3, you're driving a race car, and you're going out of your way to put in top-of-the-line fuel. Don't neglect the routine maintenance that will keep your precision machine running optimally. What's the point of being in peak physical health or having a physique that could grace the covers of fitness magazines if you're maximally stressed out, tired, angry, lonely, and unfulfilled? It's time to turn up some of those other dials.

> In the pursuit of physical optimization, **don't forget** to **enjoy your life**. Health and fitness are a means to an end, not an end in themselves. Don't let a **laser-like focus on your physique** or athletic **performance** come at the **expense** of your **mental** and **emotional health**.

As I explained in Chapter 8, sleep and stress management are important parts of overall well-being. They're not the top priorities for someone starting ADAPT Your Life Phase 1, but when you're already satisfied with your physical health, and you're not dealing with any medical conditions that are negatively affecting your quality of life, small changes to other aspects of your daily routine and general habits can have a surprising degree of impact when you want to go those last few steps. It's beyond the scope of this book to provide a detailed guide to change habits and establish new patterns, but here are some general areas for you to think about when your diet and fitness are already squared away.

Sleep

Sleep quality and quantity can affect metabolic health. Insufficient sleep and broken sleep (waking up during the night) affect hormones involved in regulating appetite and can also affect insulin sensitivity. So even when you follow a healthy diet, if you experience poor sleep, the way your body *processes* the foods you consume can be slightly different than if your sleep were on point. For someone with obesity or type 2 diabetes, the dietary shift to a very low carb intake is the most powerful step, but if you're healthy and fit, your diet is already dialed to where it needs to be. Putting some focus toward improving your sleep is a logical next step if you think this is a weak area for you.

There's no exact amount of sleep to aim for. There isn't much science behind the often-cited recommendation to get a minimum of 8 hours of sleep every night. Some people thrive on less; others need more. You can buy rings and meters and gadgets and gizmos that can measure the time you spend in various stages of sleep, and you can use these if you want—some people are enamored with the technology and can't get enough—but those tools aren't required. We've come to quantify everything—REM sleep, heart rate variability, ketone level, steps taken in a day—but the truth is that your body is the best meter you have. You probably already know whether you get enough sleep most nights or that you could be doing better. For most of us, one last social media "like" or "share" can wait until morning. That video you have to watch *now* will still be there tomorrow.

Stress

Stress management isn't much different than sleep. Most people feel a bit overwhelmed from time to time, but, as a general rule, are you able to navigate the demands of your life with ease, or do you feel like a rubber band that's pulled in a hundred different directions and is about to snap? Just like poor sleep, chronic stress negatively affects physical health. People with autoimmune conditions often experience flare-ups when they're under a lot of stress, and most of us can relate to the experience of eating a meal when feeling acute stress and then having digestive trouble—nausea, heartburn, an upset stomach.

The hormones involved in the fight-or-flight stress response raise blood sugar. In fact, that's part of what they're intended for. In modern life, you rarely encounter acutely life-threatening situations. But to your evolutionarily hardwired brain, the aggravating things you deal with often—an infuriating traffic jam, fighting with a spouse, a tight deadline at work—are no less threatening. If you were in a life-or-death situation, you would want your body to be flooded with energy so you could stay and fight for your life or run (flee) as fast as you can and get out of Dodge. The primary energy used for these intense but quick actions is glucose. Your muscles can run on fats and ketones, of course, but in emergencies, glucose is available to them much more quickly. Remember, glucose in your blood isn't the enemy. Just like insulin, you do need some glucose. What you want to avoid is too much glucose in your blood too often.

If you're chronically stressed out, your blood sugar may be a little higher than it would otherwise be. It won't be as high as if you were eating, say, donuts, fudge, or grape jam, but it could be higher than it would be if you were more relaxed. Both stress and stress relief are in the eye of the beholder. You might easily handle a situation that would immobilize someone else and vice versa. Only you know what's stressful for you, and only you know what helps you relieve stress. Some people love yoga; yoga is a *source* of stress for others. People who love to cook escape to the kitchen; those who hate it escape *from* the kitchen. There's no right or wrong approach to dealing with stress. Find what works to help *you* reframe things or to stay calm, and don't worry if it's different from what someone else would do.

Cultivate a Healthy Perspective

Human health cannot be reduced to a number on a scale, body fat percentage, mile-run time, or bench press record. No one gets a special place in history for having enviable abs. In the pursuit of physical optimization, don't forget to enjoy your life. Health and fitness are a means to an end, not an end in themselves. Don't let a laser-like focus on your physique or athletic performance come at the expense of your mental and emotional health.

Perfection sometimes comes at a cost. This cost could be neglecting important personal relationships, socially isolating yourself (passing up on engaging with friends due to uncertainty about the kind of food that will be available or opting to do a workout instead), and even weakening one of your most important relationships: the one you have with yourself. This is not a small matter. Feeling well and being able to pursue the things you enjoy are what you've earned by putting effort toward following a healthy diet and maintaining positive lifestyle habits. If you feel boxed in by fear of a dietary misstep or paralyzed by a self-imposed training schedule or some other routine, *it's okay to take a step back.*

Please don't misunderstand me here. Pursuing your personal best in whatever area of your life you're concerned with—maybe all of them—is noble, and I applaud those efforts. But total, constant perfection isn't required for feeling, looking, and performing your best. Taken too far, it can actually work against your goals. Try to maintain a healthy perspective on what you're trying to achieve. Pause now and then to reflect on whether you're getting to where you want to be, or if you're already content exactly where you are. Sometimes the grass *isn't* greener on someone else's lawn. Sometimes the best place to be is right where you are.

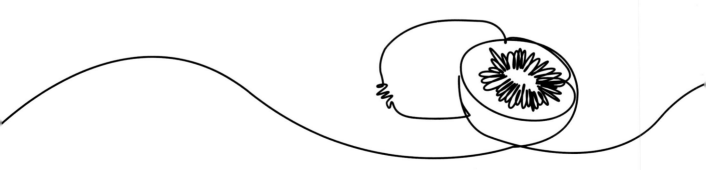

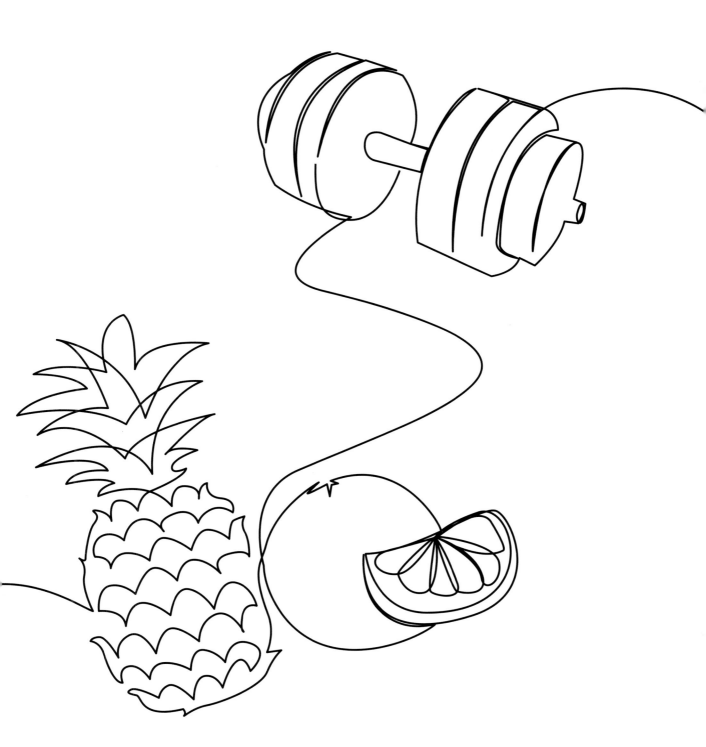

A Dedicated Athlete with Prediabetes Goes Keto, Then Increases Carbs and Continues to Thrive

"A slightly higher carb intake has allowed me to continue being competitive, train harder than ever before, and still maintain great health."

Being competitive and having a "Type A" personality has its pros and cons, and these always seem to be at war with each other. My drive and determination to compete and improve at everything I set my sights on, along with the reality that it doesn't always go my way, is a tough lesson that I've had to learn and accept through the years.

Here's an example: At the age of forty-two, I was tremendously successful in competitive sport, training, and bodybuilding. I diligently followed the best nutritional advice at the time (a high-carb, low-fat diet for more than twenty-five years). I looked great and performed well, so I assumed that the blood tests I was about to take would show outstanding health that would match my athletic performance and physical appearance. Oh boy, lesson number one...nothing could be further from the truth! You can imagine my shock when I learned that I was, in fact, prediabetic! I had a high fasting insulin and an abysmal lipid profile. What? How on Earth could this have happened to me? Well, it did. Absolutely gutted, I was determined to understand WHY. This became my immediate and obsessive focus and mission.

During this time, I came across videos on YouTube regarding the many benefits of a low-carb diet. At first, I was pretty dismissive. Years of dogma surrounding my belief that a high-carb, low-fat diet was the way to live made it difficult to accept the claims about low-carb diets. The tipping point for me was watching extremely smart doctors and researchers (people like Dr. Eric Westman, Dr. Stephen Phinney, Dr. Peter Attia, and Dr. Jeff Volek) all saying pretty much the same thing. They were not fanatical cult-like proponents of a particular narrative, but balanced, pragmatic, and completely scientific in their delivery of the facts. No hyperbole, no sensationalism. Just the data. Just the clinical results. The science was simply overwhelming, and what did I have to lose?

I set out on my journey, my very own self-experiment. At first, I embarked on a typical ketogenic protocol as defined by Dr. Eric Westman—the equivalent to Phase 1. I did this for roughly eight months. I had followed the diet faithfully and was ready to get new bloodwork and see the results of this change. I was confident I would see improvements, but I definitely wasn't prepared for just how impressive those improvements would be. My HbA1c went from 5.8 to 5.1, HDL from 61 to 108 mg/dL (1.6 to 2.8 mmol/L), and triglycerides from 141 to 62 mg/dL (1.6 to 0.7 mmol/L).

My results were amazing. However, not everything else was amazing along with them. At the time, I was a competitive cyclist and had competed as a licensed rider for around eight years. My performance in both training and racing were nowhere near where they were prior to starting keto. Standing on the podium and placing in the top five seemed to be a thing of the past. Since I wasn't overweight and no longer had any metabolic issues, I decided to adjust my carb intake. This included the timing and the selection of carbs. It's taken me seven years or so with many adjustments along the way to find my "sweet spot." This slightly higher carb intake has allowed me to continue being competitive, train harder than ever before, and still maintain similar blood markers as mentioned earlier. My current carb intake is around 80 to 120 grams total carbs on training days and around 30 to 50 grams on rest days when I don't train. I include vegetables, whole fruit, and occasionally rice and sweet potatoes in my diet. I stay away from refined sugars and typically eat fewer carbs as the day progresses.

I realize that there are many folks who are similar to me that could really benefit from my story. We are all different and all have our own journey. Luckily my journey has enabled me to continue training and competing at high levels. I am now forty-nine years old and have never felt better.

—Glen F., Cape Town, South Africa

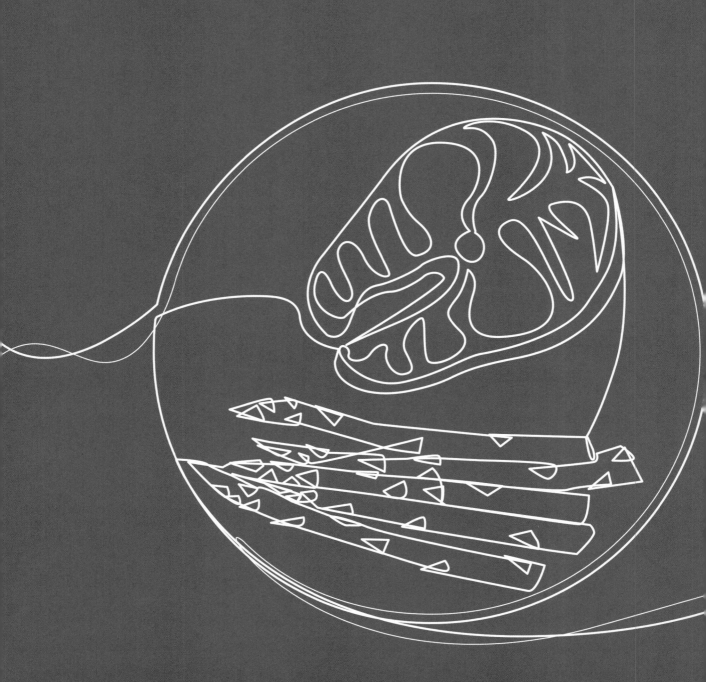

THE ADAPT YOUR LIFE DIET FOR REAL LIFE

CHAPTER 10

COURSE
CORRECTING

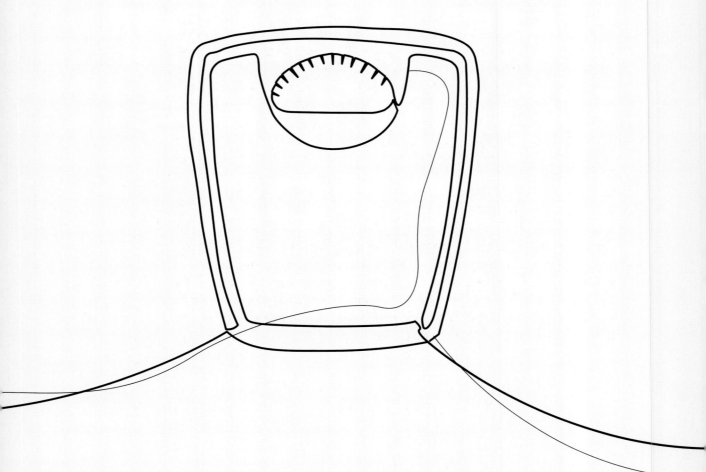

Sometimes people "graduate" from ADAPT Your Life Phase 1 to Phase 2 or from Phase 2 to Phase 3, but after a while, they start to regain some weight or discover that a health issue that had cleared up is coming back. If that happens to you, what should you do?

Simple: Return to the previous phase for a while. If you're on Phase 2, revisit Phase 1. If you're on Phase 3, revisit Phase 2. You might even choose to go from Phase 3 to Phase 1 for a total reset. If you do, you'll likely be able to make progress quickly—two weeks should be enough—so that you can move on to Phase 2. Do a pit stop there, maybe another few weeks as you gradually increase your carbs, and work your way back up to the Phase 3 amount that's best for you.

Whatever phase you were following when things started going south, assess why you experienced a setback. Were you eating more carbohydrates than you realized? Was it a stressful time for you at work or with family matters, and was your health taking a back seat? *That's okay.* Sometimes your diet isn't your top priority. Do the best you can during these times and straighten things out again as soon as you can.

You don't have to be perfect. No one is—not even the perfect-seeming diet celebrities you follow online. It's okay to stumble. You *will* stumble, in fact. You'll fall down, but you don't have to stay down. Get up and move forward. Learn from the experience so you can be better prepared to stay on plan the next time life throws you a curveball.

Above all, don't feel guilty or ashamed. Don't indulge in self-recrimination. Regaining some weight or having a health issue creep back into your life is not a sign of your failure as a person. It's helpful, in fact. Consider it educational. It's information for you to put to use so you can move forward again. If there's a pothole in the road, it's no fun driving right into it, but once you do and you know the pothole is there, you'll know to avoid it the next time you're on that road and forever after that. (But I hope your city would repair the hole eventually!)

> "Don't feel **guilty** or **ashamed** if you slip. Don't indulge in **self-recrimination. Regaining some weight** or having a health issue creep back into your life is **not a sign of** your **failure** as a person.

It's the same with stumbling a bit with your diet. If something steers you off course, learn from the experience so you'll be better equipped to manage the next time. Because, as they say, "life happens." Life *always* happens. Something will always be coming at you: financial worries, a family crisis, a burst water pipe in the middle of the night. You'll need to learn how to navigate these difficult times without medicating yourself with carbohydrates. The good news is, it won't take long before following the phase of the ADAPT Your Life Diet that's right for you is second nature, and you won't even have to think about it. You won't need to think about what to order in a restaurant or how you'll navigate Thanksgiving dinner or a work lunch.

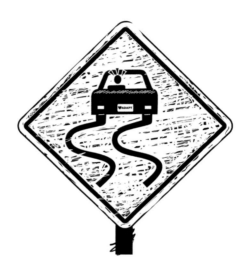

Fig 10.1: Gotten yourself a little too far off the path? No problem. A couple of wrong turns here and there don't mean you should turn around and go home. Steer yourself back to the main road and keep going!

Once you're accustomed to your new way of eating, you'll know there are always—*always*—options for you to stay on plan. If you choose not to stay on plan, then it's just that: a choice. If you take the initiative to be prepared at all times, you'll never find yourself in a situation where there is truly nothing suitable for you to eat. Keep low-sugar beef jerky in your purse or briefcase. Keep a bag of pork rinds in the trunk of your car and some canned seafood in your office desk drawer. (See Chapter 13 for suggestions for dining out and eating on the go.) And remember, if you find yourself in a situation without anything (not one thing) remotely appropriate for your phase of the diet, you might do just fine skipping a meal and "eating" your own body fat now that your body's adapted to running that way.

What If I *Really* Slip?

First, you need to determine what a "slip" is. There's a difference between having an off-plan meal once in a while and being so far off the map that you've ended up in another country. Let me start with the first scenario.

People have different names for eating off-plan. Some call it a *cheat meal*, others a *treat meal*. Whatever you call it, you're deliberately eating something you know is not the best choice for you. I don't like either of these phrases. It's not "cheating" because there's no rule book for food that you must adhere to and no laws you have to follow. Also, eating off-plan isn't much of a treat if you're eating foods that are keeping you overweight or unwell. The only person you're cheating is yourself, and that's no kind of treat.

> **Cheat meal? Treat meal?** Eating off-plan **isn't** much of **a treat** if you're eating foods that are keeping you **overweight or unwell.** The only person you're **cheating** is **yourself,** and that's no kind of treat.

People have different reasons for eating off-plan. No one reason is more or less legitimate than another when it comes to choosing to eat off-plan. Because it's just that: a choice. If you make a conscious decision to consume something you know might have negative consequences for you, take responsibility for it. Own it. You're an autonomous adult, and that means only *you* get to decide what you eat.

Earlier, I used the phrase "once in a while." If you choose to have an off-plan meal, do make it once in a while—once in a *long* while. You might find that eating a particular food once every several months is entirely worth it, or you might surprise yourself when you indulge and find that it's nowhere near as good as you remember. This experience can be disappointing, but it's also quite liberating: You won't want to eat that food anymore. If you choose to eat off-plan for a holiday meal, enjoy it with gusto and get right back to your program the next day. Don't let a holi*day* become a holi-*week* or a holi-*month*.

I recommend making off-plan meals rare and short-lived because the effects are different from the consequences of regularly straying from your carb threshold. (Really, it's best not to have off-plan meals at all, but I'm acknowledging that you're human, and there's a significant chance that you will, at some point, eat something outside of the list for your phase of the ADAPT Your Life Diet.)

One high-carb snack or meal *on occasion* won't undo all the good you've accomplished over weeks, months, or years of adhering strictly to a lower-carb way of eating, just as one Phase 1 or Phase 2 meal won't undo a lifetime of having high blood sugar or insulin. If you've been eating low-carb or keto for a while, a single higher-carb meal won't negate all the good things you've done for your body before that, in the same way that one nutritious low-carb meal doesn't negate decades of insulin resistance or high blood sugar. However, this isn't the same as saying that it's okay to indulge in high-carb foods all the time; it's a reason not to panic on the rare occasions when you do.

Ketosis Versus Fat-Adaptation

If you're following Phase 1 and you choose to measure your ketones, don't fret over getting "kicked out of ketosis" if you have a higher-carb meal. Being in a state of nutritional ketosis is not the same thing as being fat-adapted—that is, having your metabolism fueled mostly by fat so that you're no longer dependent on multiple carbohydrate-containing meals and snacks throughout the day. How do you know if you're fat-adapted? If you've been following Phase 1 or Phase 2 for a while, you're most likely there. Clues that your body is well-adjusted to running on fat include steady energy, clear thinking, and the ability to abstain from eating for several hours without craving sugar or feeling shaky, light-headed, or irritable.

> A single **higher-carb meal** won't undo all the good things you've done for your **body** before that. However, this isn't the same as saying you can **indulge** in **high-carb foods** all the time; it's a reason not to panic on the rare occasions when you do.

Ketosis is an ephemeral state. It takes very little to make it disappear—for most people, all it takes is eating just slightly more carbs than their individual threshold allows. But if you've been following a very low-carb or ketogenic way of eating for a significant length of time, then your metabolism has been adapted to running on fat for a while, and consuming slightly more carbs on rare occasion won't immediately reverse that adaptation. Just because you're not producing ketones doesn't mean you're not still fat-adapted. Fat-adaptation is hardier than the state of ketosis; it takes more to undo it. (It is possible to undo it, though! More on this in a minute.)

If you've been following Phase 1 for a while or perhaps the lower-carb end of Phase 2, then a high-carb meal will stop your body from producing ketones temporarily. However, "temporarily" is a relative term. Some people will be back in ketosis within just a few hours—as soon as their bodies have used up the glucose. For others, however—those whose bodies are particularly stubborn—it might take a few *days* to start generating ketones again.

If you don't require ketosis to feel your best, occasional higher-carb meals might be fine for you—in fact, if you're following Phase 3, they might be a regular part of your life. But if you do need to be in ketosis to have your best physical, mental, and cognitive function, then straying from your personal carb threshold will do you no favors. In fact, it will set you back. And the more often you stray, the further you'll be from where you want to go, and the longer it will take to get there.

On the rare occasions when you choose to eat a higher-carb meal, do your mental health a favor and don't weigh yourself the next day. You'll drive yourself crazy worrying about fat gain when any extra weight is actually only water. Get right back on plan, and those couple of extra water pounds will go away. (On the other hand, if seeing an abrupt increase on the scale would scare you straight and keep you from having those high-carb days too often, it might not be a bad idea to get on the scale. Know yourself and do what's best for you.)

> On the rare occasions when you choose to **eat a higher-carb meal,** do your mental health a favor and **don't weigh yourself** the next day. You'll drive yourself crazy **worrying about fat gain** when any extra weight is actually only water. Get right back on plan, and those **extra water pounds will go away.**

I said it's possible to undo fat-adaptation, so let's talk about that. Rare higher-carb meals put ketosis on hold, but they don't undo months or years of your body being adapted to running on fat. However, when higher-carb meals are more than occasional and become regular parts of your life, you will undo being fat-adapted and put yourself on a fast track to regaining weight you've lost and inviting recurrence of the health issues you have improved or put into remission.

If this starts to happen—if you regain weight or notice signs and symptoms of a health issue coming back—rein yourself in quickly and get right back on plan. If you notice your weight creeping up, it's easier to turn things around when you've regained just 8 or 10 pounds than if you've regained 80 or 100. Notice your blood sugar going back up? It's easier to nip it in the bud if your hemoglobin A1c inches up to 6.5 than if it hits 11.0. Regardless of what happens, don't let yourself feel shame and self-loathing. Learn from this valuable lesson. Listen to what your body is telling you and move forward with a stronger commitment to doing what's best for you.

Carbohydrate Addiction

I can't talk about dietary off-roading without addressing an important but perhaps uncomfortable issue. Carbohydrate addiction is real. General food addiction is real, but if you're living with a food addiction, it's most likely that you lose control over carbohydrate-containing foods—and I don't mean vegetables. Even people who aren't addicted to carbohydrates may have polished off a whole sleeve of cookies or a "family-size" bag of chips without anyone else's help. Someone who's addicted to food can and will binge on anything available, but carbohydrate-based foods tend to be the most common triggers.

So what do you do when you absolutely, positively *must* satisfy a craving? There are a few different ways to approach it, and only you know which one is best for you—and what's best might change depending on your circumstances.

Above all, know yourself. If you can have one off-plan meal or dessert on rare occasions and then get right back to your more controlled carb intake, this approach might be fine for you. As I mentioned earlier, the more often you eat off-plan, the longer it'll take for you to get the results you want. However, if these once-in-a-while dietary excursions help you stick with the ADAPT Your Life Diet over the long term, the slower pace of progress might be a trade-off you're willing to make. On the other hand, if straying from your plan for one meal or snack will make a snowflake turn into a snowball and then an all-out avalanche, you're probably better off doing everything you can to avoid getting yourself into this situation.

Again, know yourself, and don't kid yourself. There are probably some foods that you are better off abstaining from completely, forever, and there might be others that you can occasionally consume without losing control. Proceed accordingly. Although it would be best not to overeat any kind of food, if your old habits or difficult emotions are getting the best of you and you're tempted to soothe yourself with food, metabolically speaking, it's better to overconsume low-carb foods than foods that are high in sugar or starch.

When the demons are yelling in your ears, and you can't find a way to silence them, fill up on pepperoni, cheese, pork rinds, hard-boiled eggs, salami, roast beef, and other foods that are zero-carb or close to it—and don't worry about the total amount of food you're eating, even if you eat more cheese than is permitted for the phase of the diet you're following. Even if it means eating nuts when you're on Phase 1. Even if it means reaching for sugar-free chocolate or a low-carb protein bar that tastes like a cinnamon roll or a slice of birthday cake—yes, even if this bar has a high total carb count from fiber and sugar alcohols. Get through those difficult moments as well as you can by sticking as closely as possible to your food list, even if that means overeating those foods. Better to eat a large quantity of those foods than a large quantity of foods that will most certainly derail your blood sugar and insulin.

> **Know yourself,** and **don't kid yourself.** There are probably some foods that you are better off **abstaining from completely, forever,** and there might be some that you **can occasionally consume** without losing control.

Let me be clear: This advice is not for your everyday approach. It's a way to minimize the negative metabolic impact of your food choices during *rare* situations in which you find it truly impossible to stay on plan. I also want to emphasize again that when you follow the ADAPT Your Life Diet, especially Phases 1 and 2, you will find this happens less and less. It's hard to conceptualize this unless you've done it. Like giving birth or jumping out of an airplane, it's one of those experiences you can't truly understand unless you've lived it. Someone can explain it to you, and you can even watch videos of people doing it. Unless you've done it yourself, though, it's nearly impossible to understand—especially if it's radically different from anything you've experienced before. This is true of food and appetite for many people. If thoughts of food and eating have played at a constant low volume like white noise in your head for most of your life, you'll be amazed at how you feel when they *do* shut off. I can't give you an ironclad promise that this will happen for you, but it's certainly happened for thousands of my patients. (If you experience this phenomenon, come to an ADAPT Your Life event and tell your story! We'd love to have you, and you can inspire hundreds of other people. See Appendix B for information.)

Physical, psychological, and emotional addictions to food are serious matters, which is why it's important to have someone in your life who's following this plan with you. It's best if both of you start with the same phase of the diet, but even if the other person starts with another phase, they'll still be a source of moral support, encouragement, and empathy for you. Anyone can provide these things, whether they're on the ADAPT Your Life Diet or not, but having someone in your immediate family or circle of friends who understands exactly what you're going through can help you stay on plan when you're tempted to stray. There are also plenty of online forums and communities where you can find support and information from low-carb veterans who've been living reduced-carb lifestyles for years. Attending an ADAPT event is a great way to connect with other people "in real life" who are eating the way you are.

Rheumatoid Arthritis, Joint Replacements, and Limited Mobility to Low-Carb and Flourishing

"I find the low-carb, healthy-fat approach to eating extremely enjoyable, satisfying, and satiating."

I was diagnosed with first reactive then rheumatoid arthritis (RA) in 2002, at the age of 30. I lived in Germany then and ended up being quite debilitated very fast, with a high C-reactive protein (CRP, a measurement of inflammation)—more than 30 mg/L. (Less than 1 indicates very low inflammation and low risk for cardiovascular problems; between 1 and 2.9 suggests intermediate risk, and 3.0 or greater suggests a high level of inflammation.) I had lots of pain and struggled to walk and participate in daily life. I was put on three different drugs but had severe side effects, and even on the drugs, my RA was very aggressive. I had four total joint replacements (both knees and hips) between 2011 and 2013.

During this time I tried to manage my condition with supplements and saw various naturopaths and functional medicine practitioners, as well as rheumatologists. I grew increasingly dissatisfied with the lack of improvement of my condition and also the lack of understanding of RA within the medical community.

I tried all sorts of diets—vegetarian, vegan, raw food, low lectins, and more—and eventually settled on the Mediterranean diet because it seemed to have the most evidence behind it with regard to long-term health. It was also said to be anti-inflammatory. By eating mainly freshly cooked food consisting of fish, chicken, whole grains, pulses, fruit and vegetables, and very little red meat, I managed to improve somewhat, and my CRP decreased to 19. This still left me with a lot of pain, joint stiffness, and gradual destruction of my joints. Over time, my fingers started to develop severe deformities, and I struggled with loss of overall joint function, mainly in my feet, ankles, hands, and shoulders.

In 2016, my husband and I moved to the United States for two years, and during this time I started following several American health experts who happened to specialize in low-carb and ketogenic diets. I learned that this way of eating wasn't only good for weight loss but also was anti-inflammatory and showed some evidence for improving autoimmune conditions as well. This encouraged me to do my own research and then "go keto" in March 2017.

When you're having a hard time sticking to the straight and narrow, keep in mind that you may know people who could greatly benefit from following the ADAPT Your Life Diet but who feel intimidated. Leading by example is the best way to pique someone's interest. Feeling and looking your best speaks for itself, and when you stay on plan, it shows others that they can do it, too.

With full support of my husband (who is a passionate home cook), I ditched the carbs and experimented with this new way of eating. Within three weeks, I noticed various significant improvements: reduction in joint stiffness, especially in the mornings and at night, reduction of fatigue, less depression, and increased focus and mental clarity. A blood test after just six weeks of being on a strict ketogenic diet showed my CRP had dropped from 19 to 7.6. Another blood test three months later showed it had decreased even further to 4.6. Two years later, I was able to drop my pain medication and anti-inflammatories to taking just one ibuprofen a day.

I am not on a strict keto diet anymore, but I manage my condition with a low-carb, high-healthy-fat (LCHF) way of eating. It's working very well. My weight is stable and my skin and hair look great, but most importantly, my pain levels, joint stiffness, and disease activity have stayed down. While I wouldn't say that I am completely disease-free at this time, I am feeling the best I have since this all started, and gradual improvements are still coming.

I don't count any macros or calories. I find the LCHF approach to eating extremely enjoyable, satisfying, and satiating, so I don't overeat. I am never hungry, and my blood sugar is usually stable. I am a lot more focused and productive at work, too, which is an extra bonus.

What I eat a lot of: *Animal protein, like red meat, chicken, and fish (grass-fed/organic where possible), low-carb vegetables (mostly anything that's green), organic full-fat butter, goat or sheep cheese, ghee, MCT oil, avocado, home-cooked chicken or beef stock (bone broth), 90% dark chocolate.*

What I eat occasionally: *Low-carb bread (I order bread mixes online), home-baked cookies (made with butter, almond flour, coconut, and erythritol), mixed nuts, root vegetables.*

What I eat as a special treat (maybe once a month): *Pizza, sushi (with white rice), or a croissant.*

What I drink: *Coffee and black tea with added full-fat cream, green and herbal teas, and lots of water. Very occasionally I have a whiskey soda with fresh lemon or a glass of dry red wine or prosecco.*

—Sandra W., London, UK

CHAPTER 11

FREQUENTLY ASKED QUESTIONS

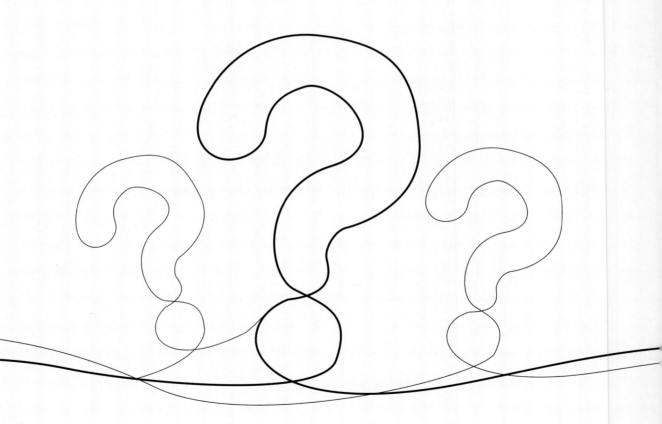

This chapter presents answers to the questions my patients ask most frequently as they start and progress through the ADAPT Your Life Diet. This resource is not intended to be a complete compendium of all possible issues you might be wondering about, but it's the core information that's most important to help you start the diet and get the results you want. Answers to advanced questions and discussions of more complex issues can be found in the videos on the ADAPT Your Life YouTube channel.

How Do I Read a Nutrition Facts Label?

Now that you know you want to focus on total carbs, how do you figure out how many total grams of carbohydrate are in a food? When looking at the label on a food package, there are two things you'll need to pay attention to: *Total Carbohydrate* and the serving size. Since the ADAPT Your Life Diet does not subtract fiber or sugar alcohols, you don't need to worry about those numbers, and you also do not need to do any math with the total sugars, added sugars, or percentages. Just look at the number of grams after Total Carbohydrate. That is the total amount of carbohydrate in one serving of the food. Next, look toward the top of the label where the serving size is listed. Since the amount of total carbohydrate listed is *per serving*, be aware of how many servings you would typically consume to see if a food is a suitable choice for the phase of the ADAPT Your Life Diet you're following. Don't accidentally sabotage yourself by consuming large amounts of a food that has only 1 or 2 carb grams per serving—if you're in the habit of eating five or six servings, you'd be consuming as much as 12 grams of total carbs.

Nutrition Facts

6 servings per container

Serving size	1 cup (230g)

Amount per serving

Calories 250

	% Daily Value*
Total Fat 12g	14%
Saturated Fat 2g	10%
Trans Fat 0g	
Cholesterol 8mg	3%
Sodium 210mg	9%
Total Carbohydrate 34g	12%
Dietary Fiber 7g	25%
Total Sugars 5g	
Includes 4g Added Sugars	8%
Protein 11g	
Vitamin D 4mcg	20%
Calcium 210mg	16%
Iron 4mg	22%
Potassium 380mg	8%

*The % Daily Value (DV) tells you how much a nutrient in a serving of food contributes to a daily diet. 2,000 calories a day is used for general nutrition advice.

Fig 11.1: A food label on a U.S. package. (Labels in other countries may provide different information.) The most important thing to look at is Total Carbohydrate. This is what you need to count on the ADAPT Your Life Diet.

Image credit: derived from maradaisy/ Shutterstock.com

In the United States, the Total Carbohydrate shown on a food label is the actual total carbs, but labels may be different in other countries. In Europe and some other parts of the world, total carbs refers to the "total glycated carbs," which is *not* the total carbs. On these labels, the fiber has already been subtracted. In these cases, you'll need to add the grams of fiber to the total glycated carbs to obtain the actual total grams of carbohydrate per serving. Also be aware that serving sizes are sometimes standardized to 100 grams of the food by weight. The amount you typically consume might be larger or smaller than this, which means the total carbohydrate you would be consuming could be higher or lower.

It might surprise you to know that if sugar appears in the ingredient list on a food label, that doesn't mean the food is automatically off-limits. (The same is true for other caloric sweeteners, like honey and molasses.) As I mentioned in Chapter 7, some of the foods permitted in unlimited amounts—such as bacon and sausage—may be cured with sugar. However, the amount remaining in the final product is close to zero, so you don't need to worry about it. (If you'd prefer to play it especially safe, seek out items that are cured without sugar. These products do exist, but they might be difficult to find because they are not available in every store.) If you are consuming very large amounts of these and you're certain you're staying within your carb threshold (by counting *total carbs*), yet you're having a hard time losing weight, consider cutting back on them and shifting toward foods that are reliably free of sugar: beef, lamb, bison, uncured pork, eggs, unseasoned chicken or turkey, and so on.

Something to be aware of is that in the United States, labeling laws allow food manufacturers to claim a product has 0 grams of carbohydrate per serving if the total amount is less than 0.5 gram. I mentioned in Chapter 8 that you don't need to stress out over fractions of a gram, but if you think you're sticking faithfully to the plan yet your results are lackluster, remember that this math is *per serving*. So if you're consuming multiple servings every day, the carbs *can* add up, and this might be what's standing in the way of your progress.

For foods that don't come with Nutrition Facts labels—for example, fresh broccoli or zucchini from your store's produce section or a farmers market—you can look up the carb counts online or—you guessed it—*stick to your list*. If you're following the guidelines for the phase of the ADAPT Your Life Diet you're on, you won't need to calculate the carbs. That's the whole point of keeping it simple.

Can I Follow the ADAPT Your Life Diet If I'm a Vegetarian?

Yes. The main issue is controlling your carbohydrate intake and avoiding sugar. These are the key principles whether you follow Phase 1, 2, or 3. If you choose to avoid consuming animal flesh, eat liberal amounts of eggs and higher-protein dairy foods, like cottage cheese and Greek yogurt. If you have a sensitivity to eggs or dairy, consider supplementing with vegetarian-friendly protein powders, such as pea protein. You'll have no trouble finding plant sources of fat: nuts and seeds, avocados and avocado oil, coconut, olive oil, and so on.

Can Children Follow the ADAPT Your Life Diet?

Yes. This plan is just food—real food: meat, poultry, seafood, dairy, eggs, vegetables, nuts, seeds, and judicious amounts of fruit and starch for those who are metabolically healthy. There is no such thing as a sugar deficiency, and no one's health—including a child's—ever got worse when they stopped eating sugar. The foods included in all phases of the ADAPT Your Life Diet provide all the nutrients children need to be healthy.

Can I Follow the ADAPT Your Life Diet If My Religion Prohibits Certain Foods?

Yes. This plan is entirely customizable. If you keep kosher, observe the laws of halal, or follow other culture- or religion-based dietary guidelines, simply consume the foods that are appropriate for your needs from the phase of the diet you're following. The foods listed are not meant as foods that you *must* consume. They are the foods you may consume at those particular carbohydrate allowance levels. From among those foods, you are free to choose the ones you enjoy and that are suitable for your life.

Can I Follow Phase 1 or Phase 2 If I Have No Gallbladder?

Yes! You might have heard that you need to follow a low-fat diet if you've had your gallbladder removed. The reason is that the gallbladder releases bile, a compound that helps break down fats so your body can digest them better. The first thing to know is that your body still makes bile even without a gallbladder; the gallbladder is just the storage sac. Your liver actually produces bile. The second thing to know is that Phases 1 and 2 of the ADAPT Your Life Diet aren't necessarily very high-fat diets. What underpins both of these phases is not keeping fat high, but keeping carbs low. That being said, you might consume more fat on Phase 1 or 2 than you were accustomed to before. If you've had your gallbladder removed or you have a history of gallstones, go easy on fat at first and increase your fat intake gradually. Loose or oily stools or an upset stomach may be signs that you're consuming too much fat in one sitting. Work with a knowledgeable doctor or health coach who can help you customize your diet and tailor your fat intake to better suit your situation. (See Appendixes A and B for resources.)

Higher-fat diets do not cause gallstones. Gallstones result from a long-term *low*-fat diet. The gallbladder *needs* fat because dietary fat is what stimulates the gallbladder to contract and release bile. When there's not enough fat in your diet, bile accumulates and stagnates in your gallbladder, eventually forming stones. If you start eating more fat, the natural, normal contraction of your gallbladder will cause the stones to dislodge and get clogged in your bile duct, triggering a gallbladder attack. Dietary fat wasn't what caused the stones to form in the first place; it was a *lack* of fat.

Can I Follow the ADAPT Your Life Diet If I Have Gout?

Yes. If you have gout, you're probably wondering if it's safe for you to consume more protein—especially red meat and seafood—which all three phases of this plan permit you to eat as much of as you want until comfortably full. As I explained in Chapter 3, gout is not caused by eating red meat or shellfish. The primary cause is chronically high insulin leading to the buildup of uric acid in the body. When your insulin level is much lower, as it will be, especially in Phases 1 and 2, your body will be better able to excrete uric acid so that it won't accumulate and form crystals in your joints, which are what's responsible for the pain and inflammation you experience during a gout attack.

Be aware, though, that if you start with Phase 1 or Phase 2 and you reduce your carbohydrate consumption very quickly—going from your usual diet to one of these very low-carb approaches overnight—you might experience some gout flares during the first few weeks or months of the transition. The reason is that uric acid competes with ketones for excretion from your body. When you are producing ketones all of a sudden, your body may prioritize excreting the ketones, leaving the uric acid behind. Your system will balance out over time, and most people with gout who adopt a low-carb or ketogenic diet find that they eventually have fewer flare-ups. Some people have none at all, even if they eat *more* red meat than before.

If you're taking medication for gout, continue taking it when you start the ADAPT Your Life Diet. As your body adjusts to your new way of eating, work with your doctor to adjust the dose or see about stopping the medicine altogether. If you're concerned about the effect of abruptly reducing your carb intake and having a gout flare, it's fine to ease into this way of eating and cut back on carbs more gradually. For example, during the first week, eliminate fruit from your diet but eat other carbs as normal (bread, potatoes, rice, beans, and so on). The second or third week, eliminate all bread and bread products. The fourth or fifth week, get rid of pasta. After that, beans and rice. Reduce your carbohydrate intake little by little until you arrive at the appropriate amount for yourself (likely Phase 1 or Phase 2). By doing it this way, you'll get to where you need to be, but your transition will be more gradual and less likely to trigger a gout flare.

What About Exercise?

As I mentioned in Part 1, exercise is great for many reasons, but losing body fat isn't one of them. You might have been exercising regularly for years, yet still had obesity or a serious health issue. That doesn't mean exercise is useless; it just means it's not that effective a tool for fat loss. To reiterate what I said in Chapter 7, I've had patients in wheelchairs or who were otherwise disabled and *couldn't* exercise, and the ADAPT Your Life Diet worked for them just as well as it did for everyone else. Being unable to exercise due to limited mobility is not an obstacle to success with this way of eating. If you have severe obesity and your mobility is hindered by your weight, joint pain, or low energy (which can affect slimmer people, too), you will likely find that both your capacity and your desire to become more physically active will increase as you lose weight—but you'll be able to lose a substantial amount without any exercise at all. The hormonal effects of carbohydrate restriction that make it easier for your body to let go of excess fat are a result of consistently lower insulin levels, and exercise is not required.

Exercise can help improve your cardiorespiratory fitness and endurance, build strength, and improve mobility, and it's good for mental health, too. These are all excellent reasons to make exercise a regular part of your life. However, what you eat has a far bigger effect on your weight than how much you exercise. Exercise because you enjoy it and it makes you feel good, not because you think it's a fast track to fat loss. And please don't use exercise to punish yourself. If you stray from your carb threshold, learn from the experience and get right back on plan. Going a little overboard on carbs is not a sin you need to atone for.

Do I Need to Take Supplements?

No. If you consume adequate foods rich in protein and fat and stick to the vegetables, fruits, and other foods on the list for your phase of the ADAPT Your Life Diet, you should not require supplementation. You may take a multivitamin if you'd like to make absolutely certain you are covering your nutritional bases. However, most of my patients take no supplements, and as long as they follow the plan laid out for them, they lose weight and experience dramatic improvements in their health without supplementing any specific nutrients. (If you are a female of reproductive age, or your doctor has told you to take iron, take a multivitamin that contains iron; otherwise, take an iron-free multivitamin.) If you're concerned that you might have shortfalls in certain vitamins or minerals, work with a doctor or nutritionist who can help identify whether this is the case and give you personalized recommendations about supplementation if warranted.

Do I Need to Fast?

No. You do not need to deliberately restrict your food intake or limit the timing of your meals. However, many people find that as their blood sugar and insulin levels are not rising and falling dramatically all day, their appetite becomes well controlled as a result. Eat when you're hungry, but you'll likely find that you're not as hungry or you don't feel hungry as often as you did when you were eating a higher-carb diet. If this means you eat only one or two meals a day, that's fine as long as you feel well and are happy with your progress.

Various fasting methods—intermittent fasting, extended fasting, time-restricted eating—have become extremely popular among people concerned about their health in general, and they've exploded onto the scene among people following controlled-carbohydrate diets. Depending on where you've previously gotten information about lower-carb ways of eating (if you've been looking), you might even think fasting is *required*. It isn't. People have been using reduced-carbohydrate diets for more than 100 years, and fasting is not necessary to be successful. Some people find that consuming all their food within a certain window of time each day (between 10:00 a.m. and 6:00 p.m., for example) and abstaining from everything but water, coffee, or tea outside that window gives them a boost in terms of clear thinking, energy level, or appetite regulation. You are free to experiment, but understand that it's not required, and you're not doing anything wrong if you don't do any kind of fasting.

That being said, keep in mind that the notion of needing three meals a day is completely artificial. Nothing at all about human physiology indicates that people must eat breakfast, lunch, and dinner, plus multiple snacks in between. Despite what you're familiar with from schools and workplaces, there's really no such thing as "lunchtime"—or breakfast time or dinnertime, for that matter. If you're hungry, eat. If you're not hungry, don't eat. Follow your appetite, not the clock.

> " There's really **no such thing** as breakfast time, **lunchtime,** or **dinnertime.** If **you're hungry, eat.** If you're not hungry, **don't eat.** Follow your **appetite**, not the clock.

Don't force yourself to go hungry, but don't force yourself to eat, either. If it's mealtime in your home, but you're not hungry, sit with your family and enjoy their company and conversation. Sip on coffee, tea, or some other noncaloric beverage if you like. You don't have to eat just because others around you are. If this makes people uncomfortable, that feeling is something for them to explore and understand about themselves: Why are they having an emotional reaction to what a grown adult is or is not eating? (I'm tempted to say it's *their* problem, not yours, but that's a little harsh. Okay, there, I said it!) You are on a journey toward better health, and being in better health—physically, mentally, cognitively—can only benefit those around you. Your family, friends, and coworkers will be the beneficiaries of your improved sense of well-being, and you can explain this to them politely and diplomatically so they'll understand why you might not be consuming food along with them at every meal.

What If My Family or Friends Don't Support Me?

Ah! A very common issue. People get awfully worked up when people close to them make life changes. A new job, a new romantic partner, a new diet: anything that threatens to change the status quo and alter relationship dynamics can make people uncomfortable. This is understandable. It's human nature, and no one is immune. If you previously went out regularly with a group of friends, they might be uncomfortable if you either opt not to join them anymore or do go but eat very differently than you ate in the past. Spouses and significant others can feel particularly threatened when a partner makes a major change—especially one that might result in significant weight loss.

There are different ways to navigate relationships when you change your diet. If friends and family are supportive, *great*. This is how it should be. The people who love you should encourage you and celebrate your victories, large and small, especially if they involve your efforts to improve your health. And remember, your whole family can do the ADAPT Your Life Diet with you, even if no one else is trying to lose weight or address a health concern. Even if they don't join you in this way of eating, you hope they'll be your cheerleaders and not your enablers.

That's an ideal situation, though. More likely, someone in your life, or perhaps multiple people, will feel so threatened by the potential changes they see in you that they'll try to sabotage you, intentionally or unintentionally. Sabotage often comes in the form of *food pushing*—"Oh, you can have just this one taste," or, "Aren't you going to have any dessert? I made your favorite!" It also comes in the form of enabling: offering you pieces of something they know you find irresistible or keeping treats in the house that they know you can't stay away from. It can even present as passive aggression—eating your favorite high-carb foods right in front of you, on purpose.

Food and eating trigger powerful feelings in people, often because those around you who are *not* making changes may feel like you're judging them, and significant others may worry that if your physique or health status changes substantially, they might not be "good enough" for you anymore. Understand that these feelings have nothing to do with you and everything to do with the person expressing them. *Their* fears. *Their* insecurity. *Their* uncertainty about how they'll fit into your life if you have a substantial transformation. They don't genuinely want to sabotage you; they're just scared. They might not even be capable of recognizing that fear is the issue, but *you* know, and now you can navigate those relationships with tact and grace.

If people close to you express negative feelings about the changes you're making, consider having a polite and calm conversation about those feelings. Let them know you understand their perspective, but make it clear that you're making these changes because you want to live a better life. If obesity or a major health issue is compromising your quality of life, then improving these things can only make you a better friend, parent, spouse, sibling, or coworker. Having a frank and honest discussion about how your health or weight is affecting you—physically and mentally or emotionally—and sharing openly with them can provide them an opportunity to do the same. Perhaps they know their own life is limited because of similar issues, but they haven't felt it was safe to be honest about it. Opening the door for this conversation can help both of you.

Eating is such a significant part of our culture. Reassure your friends and family that you can still go out with them; you're just going to be ordering differently than you were before. The food on your plate will be different, but you are the same person with the same sense of humor and the same bond, and the opportunity for good conversation and fellowship hasn't changed. If you're the primary cook in your household, it's not much different: You'll still prepare the food for the table; you'll just be avoiding the starch. If people in your life still want to interfere with you accomplishing your goals, it might be time to reassess the value of those relationships. This is easier to do with people outside your immediate family, of course. Even with relatives, though, you can take a firm but diplomatic stance. You are the only person living in your body, so you are the only one who decides what you eat.

Keep in mind that the quickest way to turn others off to this way of eating is to proselytize about it. Don't be "that person"—the one who can't eat a single molecule of food without commenting about how many carbs it does or doesn't have. Don't bring attention to what you are and are not eating, and don't sermonize about the amounts of carbs people around you are consuming. You won't want people judging you or commenting on your low-carb food selections; give them the same respect concerning the foods they eat, even if they're living with obesity or a health issue you know would be helped by carbohydrate restriction. Be the example. Stick to the program, look and feel your best, and when people start to notice how much you're changing for the better, they'll come to you to ask what you're doing.

Are Artificial Sweeteners Permitted?

Yes. In an ideal world, you would completely break your need for sweet foods, but this is a tall order. If you're dealing with obesity, diabetes, metabolic syndrome, or another cardiometabolic health issue, artificial sweeteners (sucralose, aspartame, saccharin) will be less problematic for you than regular sugar or other caloric sweeteners like honey, molasses, agave, and maple syrup. In my two decades of helping people lose weight and reverse chronic illness, I've seen thousands of patients use these sweeteners without adverse effects on their health or weight. If you can follow the ADAPT Your Life Diet without needing anything sweet, *great*. But if you can't, including artificial sweeteners can make a ketogenic or low-sugar strategy much easier to stick with over the long term—and that's what you want: Something you can do for the rest of your life, not just until your next vacation, class reunion, or some other event you want to look and feel good for. Look and feel good every day for your loved ones and for *yourself*.

Sugar alcohols and other low-carb and no-carb sweeteners, such as erythritol, xylitol, stevia, allulose, and monk fruit, are also permitted, but remember, you do not subtract sugar alcohols on the ADAPT Your Life Diet, so read labels and count the carbohydrates toward your total for the day.

What About Natural Sweeteners?

Avoid them. Sweeteners that are considered "natural," such as maple syrup, molasses, honey, and agave nectar, contain small amounts of nutrients, but ultimately, they're still just concentrated sources of sugar. If you have obesity or are living with a condition caused or exacerbated by high blood sugar or insulin, the wallop of sugar these sweeteners deliver overshadows the minuscule amount of nutrients they provide—nutrients you can get in higher amounts from other foods without the hit to your blood sugar. If you prefer to avoid artificial sweeteners *and you are metabolically healthy*, small amounts of these natural, calorie-containing sweeteners can fit into your diet.

I'm a Woman. Why Is My Husband, Brother, Father, Son, Male Coworker, or Other Man in My Life Losing Weight Faster Than I Am?

There's a joke going around: "Did you hear about the woman who went on a ketogenic diet? Her husband lost 20 pounds!" Let yourself chuckle at this joke, and then acknowledge that you're chuckling because it's true. It could be hormones, or it could be that men are generally more muscular than women, but whatever the reason, men tend to lose weight more quickly than women do, even when men aren't following the diet as strictly. This is an unfortunate phenomenon, but one that is well known among low-carb–oriented doctors and nutritionists. It's not fair, but there's not a whole lot you can do about it, so be patient with yourself, stay the course, and know that your good results will come; they'll just come a little more slowly than they do for the men in your life.

Does My Food Have to Be Organic, Grass-Fed, Pasture-Raised, and Wild-Caught?

No. This type of high-quality food can be very expensive and is out of the reach of many people. If you have the means to purchase this kind of food and you prefer to support this kind of farming, by all means, do. "Voting with your dollars" sends a powerful economic message regarding the kinds of agricultural practices and food production methods you value, and it's wonderful to support local farmers if you can. But having limited funds is in no way an obstacle to success with this way of eating. What's responsible for the metabolic effects of all phases of the ADAPT Your Life Diet is control of carbohydrate intake. As long as you stay within your carbohydrate tolerance, it doesn't matter where you buy your food or whether it is conventionally produced. You can absolutely achieve great results by sticking with conventionally produced foods purchased at your local supermarket or discount store.

Why Am I Losing So Much Hair?!

If you're looking to lose a substantial amount of weight and you stay in Phase 1 for a while, you might notice a large amount of hair loss after you've lost some weight. (This will be more obvious for women with long hair, but men and women with shorter hair may notice it, too.) I know it can be alarming to see clumps of hair coming out daily, but take it as a good sign: you're losing weight rapidly!

There's a medical term for this kind of stress-induced hair loss: *telogen effluvium*. You might not feel particularly stressed out—aside from the hair loss, you're probably feeling *great*, in fact—but this dramatic shift in your diet and the rapid fat loss it's induced is stressful to your body. But this isn't specific to Phase 1 of the ADAPT Your Life Diet or any ketogenic or low-carb diet, for that matter. It can happen any time your body goes through something it perceives

Obesity, Liver Failure, Type 2 Diabetes and a Broken Spirit to Medication-Free and Reinvigorated

"I am no longer a broken man. I have renewed hope."

We are all unique individuals. What works for me might not work for you. All I can offer you is my story and hope that it helps someone.

I came to a low-carb/keto diet for different reasons than most people. Although I had been very obese for most of my life, I had already lost 160 pounds (72 kg) prior to keto. I originally came to keto in search of help with an autoimmune liver disease (primary sclerosing cholangitis) that I was diagnosed with in November 2011. My doctor told me that most people diagnosed with this liver disease live on average eight to ten years after diagnosis. I was fifty-one at that time.

In January 2004, I spent eight days in the hospital for the third of three back and neck surgeries I'd had since 1997. This final surgery left me permanently and totally disabled at the age of forty-four. I would be unable to return to work. My father was a potato farmer and a wood contractor in northern Maine. I was fortunate that he had instilled a strong work ethic in me at a young age. I'd had different jobs over the years, all of them physically demanding in nature—I was a lumberjack and also worked in metal fabrication and as a metal machinist and welder, including helping to build battleships for the U.S. Navy. Being permanently unable to work—unable to do the backbreaking yet highly satisfying work I'd done for decades—I fell into a deep depression.

as stressful. (Sometimes it happens after a trauma or surgery, or when there are abrupt hormonal changes, such as after childbirth or during menopause.) Losing a large amount of weight relatively quickly on *any* diet, low-carb or not, can cause telogen effluvium.

The important thing to know is that your hair *will* grow back! Be patient and let your body adjust. A few months down the line, your hair will grow back, and many people report that it grows back thicker and healthier than it was before. It's a lot easier to notice your hair falling out than to notice when it starts to grow back because it can be difficult to see the tiny new growth sprouting from your scalp. Just know that what's happening is normal, and trust that your hair will grow back and fill in with time.

I was in severe pain from the combination of all my back and neck fusions. I had permanent nerve damage throughout my body and was held together with titanium rods, plates, and screws. I became addicted to painkillers because of the severe pain I was in. The type of drug I was taking is hard on the respiratory system, and being obese didn't help. (I'm 6'2" [188 cm] and weighed 330 pounds [150 kg] at the time.) I was also a very heavy smoker—up to three packs a day.

I was unable to walk on my own. I had to use a walker or cane and was able to walk only very slowly for very short distances, such as from my living room chair to the kitchen sink. In public, I needed to use a motorized scooter or cart. I was unable to lie down in a bed to sleep because of the fusions in my back and severe muscle spasms in my back and legs, which I experienced on and off all day (and continue to experience). I slept in a recliner. Despite the high doses of painkillers I was taking, the pain was still there. I had to find a way to accept that I would never be able to work again and that I could no longer do simple tasks around the house—things that healthy people do every day without a second thought.

At 330 pounds, I caused myself a hernia due to the way I had to position myself to get out of the recliner using my cane. I was scheduled for hernia surgery in April 2005. I went to the hospital for the standard presurgical blood tests, and when the results came back, the doctor said that my surgery had to be postponed: I was too sick to be operated on. My fasting blood sugar was 300 mg/dL (16.7 mmol/L), and my hemoglobin A1c was 12 percent. I had severe type 2 diabetes.

I was sent to an endocrinologist who prescribed two oral diabetes medicines and told me that eventually I would need to inject insulin because type 2 diabetes is a progressive disease. I went on to have the hernia surgery a few months later. My life continued like this for a few more years. I was fed up living this way. I knew that something needed to change—a lot needed to change.

In October 2008, I quit smoking cigarettes cold turkey. In January 2009, I quit the painkillers cold turkey. The following April, I joined a gym and started riding a recumbent bike—very slowly at first, and for only two minutes at a time. I started a daily log of my food intake and went on to lose 160 pounds (72 kg) in fifteen months. My HbA1c dropped to 6.1 percent. My doctor took me off my oral diabetes medication and told me I was no longer diabetic. (An HbA1c of 6.1 is formally classified as prediabetic.) I felt much better. I could breathe a lot easier and was able to get around more easily. My life was starting to look very different, and I started to have hope again.

I need to point out that in the course of this 160-pound weight loss, I was following a whole-food, plant-based diet. It was high in whole-food carbs, very low in fat and protein, and no red meat. I'm emphasizing this because I lost a lot of muscle mass during this time. I had lost weight and improved my health, but I still had problems and was not at my optimal potential.

In spring 2011, routine blood tests revealed abnormalities in liver function, which led to the primary sclerosing cholangitis diagnosis. Being diagnosed with a fatal liver disease hit me with full force. My doctor told me that this condition had no known cure and no effective treatments. Essentially, I was sent home to die. I got knocked down, but I didn't stay down. I started researching autoimmune diseases, liver diseases, and diabetes. I spent a year researching and studying before starting a very-low-carb, adequate-protein ketogenic diet, combined with intermittent fasting and exercise in November 2012.

Because of the diagnosis, I had liver function tests done every six months. The re-sults slowly began improving, with dramatic improvement after eighteen to twenty-four months on keto. Today my liver function tests are those of a healthy person with no disease, and I get the bloodwork done only once a year. My lipid panel (cholesterol and triglycerides) is excellent, and my HbA1c has been between 4.8 and 4.9 percent for the last seven years—all without any diabetes medications, only diet and exercise.

I have finally found peace with myself. I have accepted the fact that I will never be able to work again, but I am no longer a broken man. I have renewed hope—hope that I will live long enough to watch my grandchildren grow into adulthood.

—Jeff C., Brunswick, Maine

CHAPTER 12

MEAL AND SNACK IDEAS

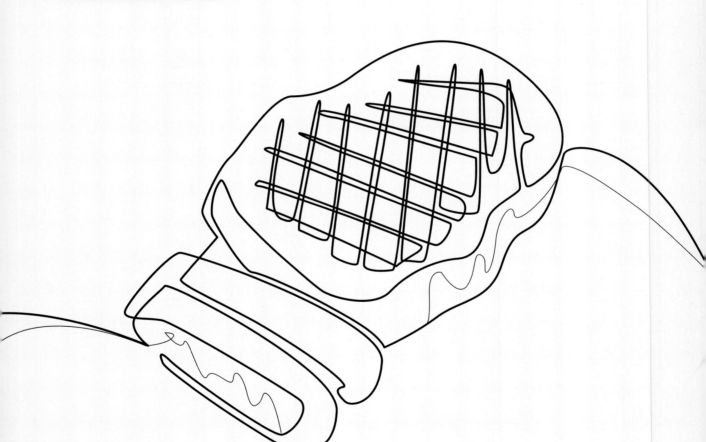

Thanks to creative cookbook authors and bloggers, there's a world of cookbooks, apps, and recipe websites that are suitable for all three phases of the ADAPT Your Life Diet. Choose recipes that contain ingredients that fit within your carb threshold or customize them as necessary. Look at keto cookbooks for recipes that are better suited for Phase 1 and keto and low-carb cookbooks for Phase 2 or 3. Cookbooks geared toward Paleo-style diets are fine for the higher-carb end of Phase 2 and Phase 3. (Many Paleo recipes are low-carb or even keto, but some contain potatoes, carrots, beets, parsnips, and other sweet or starchy foods that are best suited for Phase 3.)

If you're following Phase 1, be careful with recipes you choose that are labeled as "keto" because many will be very high in fat. This is fine, but if you're struggling to lose body fat, stick to recipes that are somewhat lower in fat or decrease the amount of fat called for if it won't alter the final dish too much. Remember, even when your carbohydrate intake is very low, fat is not unlimited if you're trying to lose a substantial amount of weight. Going overboard on fat (especially from added fats such as heavy cream, cheese, butter, and oils) often makes it more difficult for some people to lose body fat even when carbs are low.

Whatever cuisines you like most, you will have no problem finding appropriate recipes. There are keto, low-carb, and Paleo cookbooks and recipe websites for Mexican, Middle Eastern, Mediterranean, East Asian, Indian, and many other kinds of food. You even can find recipes to replicate fast-food favorites. There are cookbooks specifically for slow cookers and pressure cookers, and these tools can make the ADAPT Your Life Diet a cinch to stick to—advance preparation is the name of the game. Cook a multi-pound roast or another large piece of meat in a slow cooker or pressure cooker and eat from it for days. This goes for single people, too: just because you're cooking for one doesn't mean you can't prepare a 3- to 4-pound piece of meat; it'll feed you for days.

What to Eat

Honestly, you can eat anything you like, as long as you stick to the food list for the phase of the diet you're following. You are free to experiment with including other foods if they fit within your carbohydrate threshold, but I cannot guarantee you'll get the same results that you would by sticking strictly to the foods on the list.

People often ask me for meal plans or recipes, but I'd prefer you discover how easy it is to eat the ADAPT Your Life way *without* a plan. If you keep your fridge, freezer, and pantry or cupboards stocked with ingredients that are suitable for your phase of the diet, you'll be able to put meals together in minutes.

> The **ADAPT Your Life Diet** is just **regular food.** The only thing that's changing from your existing diet is the **amount of carbohydrate** you'll be eating.

Something to keep in mind when thinking about what you'll eat is that there's no such thing as "breakfast food," "lunch food," or "dinner food." Most of us are accustomed to thinking of eggs, bacon, sausage, cereal, toast, or bagels when it comes to breakfast, but in many parts of the world, breakfast is just a meal, no different from lunch or dinner, and people don't consume specific foods in the morning. Outside North America, it's not uncommon to have meat or fish and vegetables for breakfast.

The same goes for lunch: No laws state that you must eat a sandwich in the middle of the day. Like breakfast, lunch is just a meal—an opportunity to give yourself nourishment, which can come in the form of any food you like, as long as you stay within your carb threshold. As for dinner, well, you might turn things upside down and have an omelet for dinner. Nothing wrong with that! Separate yourself from the idea that specific foods are best suited for certain meals. Food is food, regardless of the time of day you eat it, and regardless of whether you eat one, two, or three meals a day. The ideas in the following sections aren't specifically for breakfast, lunch, or dinner; they're just to get you thinking about the kinds of foods and food combinations you can enjoy while following the ADAPT Your Life Diet approach, and they're fine for any time of day.

Even if you don't normally follow specific recipes, I recommend looking at keto, low-carb, and Paleo cookbooks and recipe websites to get ideas and inspiration for possibilities you might not have thought of. But don't forget: the ADAPT Your Life Diet is just regular food; the only thing that changes from your existing diet is the amount of carbohydrate you'll be eating.

ADAPT Your Life Phase 1

You might think Phase 1 is nothing but bunless bacon cheeseburgers and salads with no croutons. If it were, there'd be nothing wrong with that, but the truth is, you can enjoy a world of variety on Phase 1 whether you prefer gourmet meals made from scratch or a simple meal of a can of tuna with a little mayo mixed in and some cucumbers and celery on the side.

Since there are no grains on Phase 1, bread, buns, pita, wraps, tortillas, and anything else you commonly put meat or vegetables into are off limits. Use lettuce or cabbage leaves as a substitute, or better yet, just get used to eating with a fork and knife. Here are some ideas for Phase 1 meals and snacks, but you can eat *any* combination of foods prepared any way you like, as long as you stay within the food list!

- Broiled salmon with asparagus and hollandaise sauce
- Canned salmon or mackerel with sliced raw green pepper, cucumber, or mushrooms
- Fajitas, minus the tortillas/wraps (chicken, beef, shrimp, onions, and peppers)
- Bunless burger, cheeseburger, or turkey burger with the works—bacon, lettuce, onion, tomato, pickles
- Deviled eggs prepared any way you like as long as the ingredients are within your carb threshold
- Roast beef or turkey roll-ups: sliced deli meat spread with a thin layer of cream cheese or guacamole topped with chopped scallion or a strip of sliced green pepper and rolled up (use garlic and herb cream cheese for extra flavor)
- Frittata or crustless quiche: eggs, cream, cheese, onion, spinach, and mushrooms
- Pork loin or beef roast in slow cooker or pressure cooker with Phase 1 vegetables (serve with mashed cauliflower or cauliflower rice)
- Stuffed peppers without rice—just meat and sauce or add diced peppers and onions
- Steak, pork chops, or roast chicken with roasted Brussels sprouts and/or radishes
- Egg salad, tuna salad, or chicken salad in lettuce wraps or simply eaten with a fork
- Cobb salad (iceberg or romaine lettuce, grilled chicken, hard-boiled egg, crumbled bacon, blue cheese, and avocado)

- Grilled sausage and peppers
- Meatballs with zucchini noodles and tomato sauce
- Chili with cubed or ground beef or bison, chicken or turkey, canned tomatoes, onions, peppers, and whatever sugar-free seasoning you like. (No beans.)
- Pork rinds dipped in guacamole or cream cheese– or sour cream–based dip
- Cauliflower crust or meat crust pizza (find recipes online)
- Antipasto spread with cheese, olives, cured meats, marinated mushrooms, and artichoke hearts

ADAPT Your Life Phase 2

The ideas suitable for Phase 1 still work, plus these suggestions:

- Entrée salad with mixed lettuce, grilled chicken or steak, crumbled blue cheese or feta, shredded carrots, and sliced mushrooms
- Grilled pork chops with mashed turnips
- Meatballs and sauce over spaghetti squash
- Roasted turkey breast with carrots, onions, and fennel
- Lamb stew or tagine with butternut squash
- Plain yogurt topped with raspberries or blackberries
- Roasted beet and goat cheese salad (great with arugula)
- Greek mezze platter: olives, halloumi cheese, marinated grilled chicken and vegetables (onions, zucchini, yellow squash), homemade or store-bought tzatziki sauce
- Low-carb cracker or crispbread with cream cheese or cold cuts
- Pad Thai with zucchini noodles
- Cottage cheese topped with cinnamon and chopped toasted pecans, walnuts, or almonds
- Shrimp and vegetable stir-fry (onions, snow peas, bell peppers, broccoli, carrots)
- Lasagna with ground meat, ricotta cheese, and tomato sauce (substitute thinly sliced zucchini for pasta sheets)

ADAPT Your Life Phase 3

Enjoy anything suitable for Phases 1 and 2, plus the following suggestions:

- Slow-cooked pork or beef roast with roasted root vegetables (sweet potato, beets, parsnips, carrots)
- Grilled steak with baked or mashed potatoes or sweet potatoes
- Roasted chicken over rice
- Chili with beans
- Seafood risotto
- Cold pasta salad with pesto sauce, chicken, and pine nuts
- Vegetable crudités with hummus (can include pita bread or chips)
- Niçoise salad, which is tuna or salmon, butter lettuce, green beans, soft-boiled egg, olives, boiled fingerling potatoes or other lower-starch potato, and anchovies (if desired)
- Stuffed peppers (may include rice, if desired)
- Pork chops or pork loin with apples
- Fruit salad topped with unsweetened shredded coconut and sliced almonds

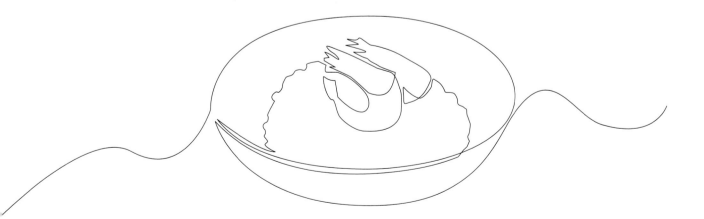

No Meal Plans?! No Recipes?!

Nope. I don't give you meal plans or recipes, and here's why. The ADAPT Your Life Diet is infinitely customizable. You can construct your diet entirely from restaurants and fast-food joints or cook every meal at home from scratch. Whether your cooking skills extend solely to opening cans and pressing buttons on a microwave or your kitchen is stocked with all the latest gadgets and gear, you'll be able to enjoy a world of different foods while reaping the metabolic and health benefits of any phase of the diet.

> " People often ask me for meal plans or recipes, but I prefer you **discover how easy** it is to eat **the ADAPT Your Life** way **without** a plan.

Think of it this way: if you were a freelance artist—a writer, a painter, a sculptor—working on a project with a deadline, the person you're working for doesn't care when or how you do the work as long as the project is completed before the deadline. You could work on it in your pajamas or wearing a business suit. You could spend time on it at 2:00 a.m. or 4:00 p.m. As long as you make the deadline, you have total freedom as to when and how you get the work done. With the ADAPT Your Life Diet, as long as you stick to foods on the list for your phase and stay within the recommended amounts, what you choose to eat is flexible. Don't like broccoli or kale? Choose different vegetables. Not a fan of fish? Skip seafood and get your protein from other sources. The ADAPT Your Life Diet is a framework—a set of guidelines—not a set of commandments carved in stone.

Remember, the ADAPT Your Life Diet is about food—no special shakes or soups, no magical concoctions that cost a small fortune. Phases 1 and 2 include foods you've been eating all your life, minus all or most of the sugar and starch. Phase 3 allows for substantially more carbohydrate, but as you can see from the ideas I shared, the foods you'll be eating on Phase 3 aren't foreign at all—steak and a potato, chicken with rice. If you'd like to branch out and explore specific recipes, as I previously mentioned, there are numerous low-carb and keto cookbooks and recipe websites. You'll have no problem finding a multitude of suitable dishes.

Batch Cooking

Go big or go home. The number one tip that can make the ADAPT Your Life Diet a breeze is *leftovers*. In most cases, it doesn't take more time to cook a large amount of food than it does to cook a small amount, so you might as well make a large amount. If you're going to cook something, cook a lot of it, especially if you don't enjoy cooking and wouldn't want to do it every day. Even if you do love to cook, you'll no doubt have days when you are pressed for time or have a last-minute schedule change, and your cooking time disappears. Having food prepared in advance will make it much easier to stick to your program no matter how busy you are or what life is throwing at you. And the best time to prepare food is when you're *not* hungry.

Hard-boiled eggs: Hard-boiled eggs can be your best friend for a quick, convenient, and portable source of protein and fat. They can be a snack or a meal, or later in the week, you can turn them into egg salad. If you're boiling eggs, why boil only two or three? Boil two *dozen*. They'll last for up to a week in the fridge, and they're perfect for all three phases of the diet.

Chicken breasts, thighs, or leg quarters (with or without skin and bones): If you're cooking chicken, go ahead and cook two or three packages at once using your preferred cooking method (grilled, roasted, baked, broiled). You can use the cooked chicken for a meal on the day you cook it or cut the pieces into strips or chunks and eat them cold as a snack or meal some other time. (They'll be great dipped in blue cheese or ranch dressing or guacamole). You also can use cooked chicken as the protein in a lunch or dinner salad or reheat it as part of chicken chili, fajitas, or even an omelet or frittata.

Steak: Never cook just one steak. Like I've said, if you're grilling or broiling anyway, you might as well cook several steaks at once. Have one for dinner and slice another to use in a salad the next day or the day after that. You can also treat yourself to steak and eggs one morning, or as I suggested for the chicken, make an omelet, frittata, or fajitas. (This tip applies to pork chops or grilled or roasted pork loin, too.) Sliced cold steak is a perfectly fine snack either by itself or dipped in blue cheese dressing, mayo, or a sour cream–based dip. Cold steak is a zero-carb, high-protein choice suitable for all three diet phases.

Sausages and bacon: Cook large batches of sausage and bacon. Cold bacon or sausages make excellent snacks or on-the-go breakfast. Zip-top bags and reusable plastic containers are your friends. Another use for precooked bacon is to crumble the bacon on a salad or top a bunless burger with it.

Raw vegetables: Wash, peel, slice, or dice raw vegetables and keep them stored properly in the fridge. Having good food in your home does you no good if you don't actually eat it, and you're more likely to eat vegetables if the time-consuming preparation is already done so all you have to do is reach for the container. When you come home from the store or farmers market, put on some good music and take a little time to prep everything so it's ready when you need a snack.

Cooked vegetables: Roast, steam, grill, bake, or sauté a large quantity of vegetables at once. Use them as side dishes; in salads, omelets, or crustless quiches; or as a snack by themselves. Steam a pile of broccoli, cauliflower, or zucchini and leave it plain—no sauce, no seasoning. Then, you can use it any way you like later in the week: tossed into a stir-fry, eaten cold as a snack, blended into a soup, and so on.

Big-batch soups and entrées: Prepare dishes that are typically intended to be made in big batches: think chili, stews, soups, curries, and stir-fries. You can cook one time and then serve yourself meals for a few days in a row. If you prefer, eat some for a day or two and put the rest in the freezer for a day when you don't feel like cooking. A slow cooker or pressure cooker is helpful for cooking large batches. Large roasts are also good for big-batch cooking: Cook a large beef roast, pork shoulder, or similar cut of meat. You can reheat it over the next few days or eat it cold—cold, sliced roast beef with horseradish sauce is a dynamite low-carb treat.

Lifelong Athlete with Prediabetes and High Blood Pressure Regains Health with Low-Carb

"I love the food I'm eating and cooking, and I feel amazing."

I am a fifty-two-year-old black female who has been active and fit her entire life. I grew up playing soccer and basketball, and I ran track. I was a Division I collegiate soccer player and played semi-professional soccer. I hike, bike, run, swim, and more. My weight has always been within a range of 10 or so pounds, with the highest in college (145 to 150 pounds [66 to 68 kg]) and after college and through my mid-forties (135 to 140 pounds [61 to 63 kg]).

I was raised on a standard American (high-carb) diet and continued to eat this way into adulthood. I always thought I could maintain my weight by exercising more and eating less: calories in versus calories out. And for me, with regard to my weight, this seemed to work. I never dieted, per se, just "moved more." My diet was pretty varied from real whole food to processed junk. Breakfast ranged from toaster pastries to

Defrost! All the great food you prepare ahead of time and freeze does you no good if you've just gotten home from work, the family's hungry, and nothing is defrosted. This is where you may need a little planning and forethought—defrost something overnight so it's ready to go the next day, or better yet, always, *always* have something high in protein and fat in the fridge ready to be cooked, such as a pound of ground beef (or several pounds, depending on how many people you're feeding) or some chicken thighs. Most cuts of meat take only minutes to cook if they're already defrosted. Get in the habit of keeping a few pounds of ground meat, loose sausage, chicken legs, or similar meats in your fridge at all times.

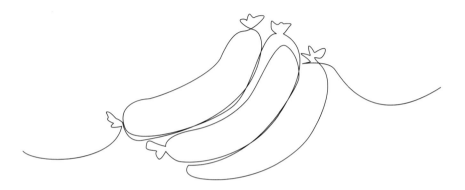

steel-cut oatmeal. During hikes, I would munch on energy bars and granola with dried fruit. My favorite snacks were gummy worms and kettle-cooked potato chips. I enjoyed desserts, ice cream, cakes and pies, as well as wine, beer, and the occasional mixed drink. My favorite beers were the microbrews, lots of hops, a high alcohol content—and lots of carbs, I know now.

I am the most fit person in my family. Most of my relatives have some component of metabolic syndrome, and my family history includes type 2 diabetes, hypertension, heart disease, obesity, dementia, and cancer. My father has hypertension and central obesity, and he had a heart attack at age sixty. He was recently diagnosed with vascular dementia (possibly Alzheimer's disease) and has severe arterial calcification. My older brother had colon cancer at the age of forty-six. He also has type 2 diabetes and was diagnosed with congestive heart failure at age fifty-five.

The women in my family have not fared any better. Breast cancer runs in my family, with my maternal grandmother and maternal aunt both having the disease and dying from a perforated colon and a massive heart attack at ages fifty-nine and sixty-eight, respectively. My maternal aunt also lived with type 2 diabetes for most of her life. My mom is seventy-five and was diagnosed with early onset dementia at age sixty-eight. She also has hypertension and central obesity. I was hoping to avoid all this and trusted that my active lifestyle would get me through my forties, fifties, and even my sixties free from chronic disease.

I wasn't so lucky. By my late forties, my blood pressure and blood sugar were increasing. My hemoglobin A1c was 5.7 (in the prediabetes range). My blood pressure was in the prehypertensive range. Fearing that my blood pressure would continue to rise until I reached full-blown hypertension, I asked my doctor if I could go on a low dose of blood pressure medicine. I also asked my doctor about the 5.7 A1c measurement to see what I could do to lower it. My doctor was not very concerned since the range was at the very low end of prediabetes. I wasn't overweight, and I was very active, so the doctor said I shouldn't worry. However, knowing my family history made me worry, so I turned to the internet to see how I could lower my blood sugar and my blood pressure.

My brother went vegan after his colon cancer treatment and suggested that I try it. I followed a vegan diet for about four months in the fall/winter of 2016. I love to cook and I enjoyed making the imitation cheese and meat products using plant ingredients. At the time, I was hoping this animal-free way of eating would lower my blood pressure. During this time, I lost weight, my blood pressure was still controlled with the medication, and my cholesterol decreased significantly, but my A1c actually increased: up to 5.8. I came across a popular low-carb website, where I read everything they published and signed up for a membership. I also reviewed my old biochemistry lessons. (I have a master's degree in nutritional biochemistry from NC State.)

I decided to start eating keto in January 2017 and have not looked back. I love the food I'm eating and cooking, and I feel amazing. I know the science, and avoiding grains, processed foods, seed oils, and sugar are not a problem for me. I've even given up the *beer and have reduced my wine consumption and frequency. My blood pressure nor-malized, so I was able to stop the medication. After only six months, my A1c dropped to 5.3, and today it's 5.1—completely normal and far below the threshold for prediabe-tes. I'm at my lowest weight since high school. I am lean and strong, and I have tons of energy. I practice good sleep hygiene and wake up refreshed. I routinely work out in the mornings before even eating anything, and I feel amazing.*

In the beginning of keto, I set and tracked my macros using an app. I kept my net carbs between 20 and 40 grams. There were some days that I was in the ketogenic range and others where I was low-carb. Also in the beginning, I really watched my protein intake, eating around 90 grams a day. I don't worry about how much protein I get now, though, and usually base my meals around my protein source. I also drank fatty coffees and made "fat bombs." Now I drink my coffee black with salt and collagen powder (for my joints). I make keto breads and sweets using ingredients I know work for me. I really don't add much extra fat to my food. I eat the fat that comes along for the ride already as part of the food.

Keto/low-carb has been an amazing gift to my health. I know that there are no guar-antees in life, but I think by eating keto/low-carb, I am stacking the deck in my favor to remain healthy and free of many of the diet-driven diseases. I am so thankful for social media. Without low-carb and keto information from Facebook, Twitter, and YouTube, I would still be taking blood pressure medicine and likely would be on my way to diabetes and memory loss.

—April K., Chapel Hill, NC

CHAPTER 13

FOLLOWING THE ADAPT YOUR LIFE DIET WHEN DINING OUT OR EATING ON THE GO

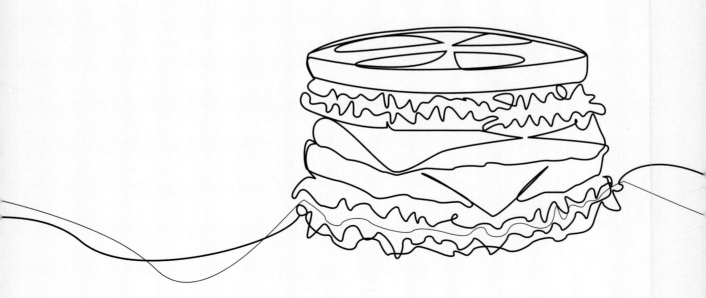

If you enjoy dining out, you'll have no problem continuing to do so while following any phase of the ADAPT Your Life Diet. Ask for appropriate substitutions for higher-carb items, and you'll be able to find plenty of dishes suitable for you no matter where you are or what kind of restaurant you visit. "There was nothing I could eat!" is not a valid excuse for throwing caution to the wind. Armed with the advice in this chapter, you will always be able to find food that works for you, whether you're following Phase 1, Phase 2, or Phase 3.

As food allergies become more common and people become more health-conscious, variations of lower-carb, ketogenic, and Paleo-style diets have become more popular, and restaurant servers and chefs are not put off or surprised by special requests. In fact, many restaurant menus now specifically feature low-carb or keto-friendly dishes, which helps take the guesswork out of things for you. Servers will not look at you funny if you ask them not to bring the bread basket and to leave the bun off your burger.

General Principles

Here are some tips for selecting dishes that will enable you to stay on-plan and continue getting the benefits of your way of eating. The following suggestions are best for Phases 1 and 2. If you're following Phase 3, your carbohydrate intake is more liberal, and you will have more flexibility to partake of potatoes, beans, rice, and so on. Order accordingly.

- Choose dishes that are prepared *simply*: Grilled, baked, steamed, or roasted meats, poultry, seafood, nonstarchy vegetables, and salads are good go-to items. Fried foods are best avoided—not because frying is a problem (no need to fear fat anymore), but because fried foods are most likely coated in flour-based breading or batter, which will take a zero-carb food like chicken or fish and turn it into a higher-carb food. If there's a sauce that includes ingredients you're not sure of, ask the server to tell you what's in it. Many sauces contain sugar, corn syrup, corn starch, and/or flour. This is why it's best to stick with dishes with simple preparations.

- Avoid all pasta, rice, bread, noodles, potatoes, corn, beans, sugar-sweetened soda, desserts, and obvious sources of sugar and starch.

- Be careful with condiments. Ketchup is relatively high in carbs, and many salad dressings contain large amounts of sugar or corn syrup. Your best bets for condiments are mustard (any kind except honey mustard), mayonnaise, hot sauce, melted butter, olive oil, vinegar, and dressings that are typically very low in carbs, such ranch, blue cheese, or Caesar. (Take some time to look at labels in supermarkets to get an idea of which types of dressings are lowest in carbs so you'll know what to ask for at a restaurant. Carb counts per 2-tablespoon serving should be 2 grams or less.)

- At restaurants where free bread or rolls are provided before the food is served, request that the wait staff not bring those to the table. Ask for something else if it is the type of restaurant that is likely to have something available; for example, sometimes olives or pickles can be served instead of starches and grains. If you're dining with others who are not restricting their carb intake, you might just have to wait patiently while they eat the bread. Enjoy the wait—your steak, chicken, pork chop, shrimp scampi, or cobb salad is going to be delicious, and it'll be even more so if you're a tad hungrier when it arrives.

- Ask for a double portion of nonstarchy vegetables in lieu of a starchy side dish—for example, a double serving of broccoli instead of a potato or roasted vegetables instead of pasta or rice. You might also be able to substitute a salad for a starchy item. Some restaurants will charge a small fee for this. It's unfair, but you are worth the extra couple dollars!

- Prepare ahead of time. Many restaurants post their menu online. Review it to see what will be suitable for you, and you'll have an easier time ordering. If necessary, you can suggest a change of venue.

Tips for Specific Cuisines

No matter what type of cuisine you prefer, it's easy to customize your order to make your meals suitable for any phase of the ADAPT Your Life Diet. It may be hard to imagine Asian food without noodles and rice or Italian minus pasta and bread, but as you'll see, simple swaps and substitutions will allow you to continue enjoying your favorite restaurants while experiencing the benefits of lower-carb eating.

- **Mexican:** Fajitas are an ideal choice because they're just grilled meat and vegetables, and you can enjoy sour cream, cheese, guacamole, and salsa as condiments. Ask the server to hold the tortillas and bring extra vegetables instead of rice and beans. At some fast-food Tex-Mex chains, you can get meat, lettuce, cheese, and vegetables in a lettuce bowl instead of a flour or corn wrap, which is a slam dunk for a low-carb diet!

- **Middle Eastern/Greek:** Choose kebabs or other grilled-meat dishes. Ask for extra vegetables or meat instead of rice or pita bread. Avoid hummus, stuffed grape leaves (which contain rice), and anything else with beans or high starch. These cuisines are famous for grilled meats; take advantage of this, as well as marinated feta cheese, olives, and seared halloumi cheese. Keto perfection.

- **Indian/Afghan/Pakistani:** These cuisines are somewhat similar to Middle Eastern and Greek cuisines. Avoid rice, pita bread, naan, chickpeas, and potatoes. Instead, choose curries and dishes of grilled or roasted meat and vegetables. Curries may be thickened with corn starch or another carb-based item, but the total amount of carbs in your meal will be very low if you avoid the obvious sources of starch and sugar. Remember, the ADAPT Your Life Diet is not about perfection; it's about doing the best you can under the circumstances you find yourself in.

- **Barbecue:** A good BBQ restaurant is a carbohydrate-restrictor's best friend! Any cut of meat is fine if it's cooked without sauce: beef brisket, pulled pork, smoked chicken, ribs, sausages, etc. Avoid bread, cornbread, and sweet or starchy sides (mac and cheese, baked beans, hush puppies). Instead, opt for collard greens, green beans, or any other nonstarchy side dish—but it's okay to skip the vegetables altogether and fill up on the meat. That's why you go to a barbecue restaurant! Avoid BBQ sauces unless you know they're sugar-free. (This is rare in restaurants, but you can make your own at home.) Most sauces are primarily corn syrup. If the meat is cooked right, you won't need sauce anyway. Don't worry about dry rubs that might have been used on the meat. The total amount of sugar remaining in the final dish will likely be very low, and you'll steer clear of the majority of the carbs by skipping the starchy sides and sweet sauces.

- **Chinese/Japanese/Thai:** East Asian cuisines can be difficult to make low-carb, but it's not impossible. Ask for your dishes to be prepared *steamed* or with *no sauce* because sauces typically contain sugar and corn starch. Use soy sauce or hot mustard as condiments. Good choices for Chinese takeout are steamed chicken or shrimp with mixed vegetables. Some restaurants also offer grilled chicken or beef on skewers. Avoid rice, noodles, wontons, dumplings, deep-fried foods, egg rolls, spring rolls, and tempura (due to the wraps and breading). Sashimi is perfect; just avoid sushi rice. For Thai restaurants, avoid noodle and rice dishes. Choose curries that contain meat or seafood and vegetables, spices, and coconut milk.

- **Italian:** Pasta is off-limits during Phases 1 and 2, but most Italian restaurants have other options that are perfect for low- and very-low-carbohydrate diets. Choose salads, steaks, chicken, pork chops, or seafood with vegetables. Avoid bread and breadsticks, and ask for no croutons on your salad. Ask for extra nonstarchy vegetables instead of pasta or potatoes as side dishes. If there's an antipasto appetizer (cured meats, cheese, olives, marinated vegetables), go for it! You might even be able to order a larger portion as an entrée.

- **Diner/Bistro/Pub:** These types of restaurants typically have diverse menus, and finding suitable options will be easy. Use the same logic as for any other restaurant: no grains or other starchy carbohydrates and no sweets for dessert. Cobb, chef, and Caesar salads are good choices (no croutons). Burgers and sandwiches without buns or bread are reliable go-tos, as are steaks, pork chops, or grilled chicken with nonstarchy vegetables. Always ask for nonstarchy vegetables instead of fries or other potato sides. You can often substitute a simple house salad for a starchy side dish. Other good selections include any type of roasted meat, poultry, or fish, or a platter of egg or tuna salad on a bed of lettuce.

- **Breakfast:** Stick with eggs, bacon, ham, sausage, and other items you know are low in carbs. Avoid pancakes, waffles, potatoes, toast, bagels, muffins, fruit, juice, and jam/jelly. Western omelets are a great option (eggs, ham, onion, peppers), as is any type of omelet that contains eggs, meat, cheese, and/or low-starch veggies (peppers, spinach, mushrooms, onions, zucchini). Any other eggs are fine, too: poached, scrambled, over-easy, hard-boiled—however you prefer them. Use mustard, mayonnaise, or hot sauce as condiments.

- **Entrée Salads:** Customize salads as necessary: no dried fruits, fresh fruit, crunchy noodles, or other sweet or starchy add-ons. Stick with lettuce, spinach, and other greens. Suitable additions include chopped hard-boiled egg, bacon, cheese, avocado, ham, turkey, chicken, steak, salmon, olives, cucumbers, sliced peppers, radishes, and other nonstarchy vegetables. Use oil and vinegar or a high-fat dressing like ranch or blue cheese. Avoid thousand island, French, honey mustard, raspberry vinaigrette, and other sweetened dressings. (For Phases 2 and 3, you can include carrots, beets, sunflower seeds, sliced almonds, or other nuts and seeds.)

Eating on the Go or on the Road

Just as with dining out, you will have no trouble finding suitable options to eat if you're on the road frequently or a hectic schedule has you running from one task to the next without time to prepare food or sit down to a full meal. Being pressed for time or being away from your usual cooking environment doesn't need to be an obstacle to sticking with any phase of the ADAPT Your Life Diet. Low-carb foods are increasingly available just about everywhere, so you'll be able to find something great no matter where you are.

Foods to grab from a quick run into a grocery store:

- Salad bars enable you to customize according to your phase of the diet: lettuce, peppers, mushrooms, olives, chicken, ham, bacon, turkey, tuna, cheese, radishes, hard-boiled eggs, and cucumbers. Add carrots, beets, nuts, seeds, and beans as appropriate for Phase 2 or 3.

- Antipasto bar: olives, cheese, marinated mushrooms, artichoke hearts, salami or other cured meats.

- Cold cuts and cheese, which you can find either prepackaged or select from the deli counter.

- Rotisserie chicken or turkey breast.
- Tuna, salmon, mackerel, or sardines in pouches or pop-top cans.
- Pepperoni or salami sticks.
- Deli department prepared egg salad or tuna salad.
- Pork rinds and guacamole.
- Nuts (for Phase 2 or 3): plain, salted, or unsalted, but avoid honey roasted.

Foods to grab at a gas station or convenience store:

- Hard-boiled eggs
- String cheese, cheese sticks
- Packets of cream cheese
- Beef jerky: plain or original flavor because BBQ, teriyaki, and others have more sugar
- Pork rinds
- Pepperoni
- Hot dogs without buns
- Nuts (for Phase 2 or 3)

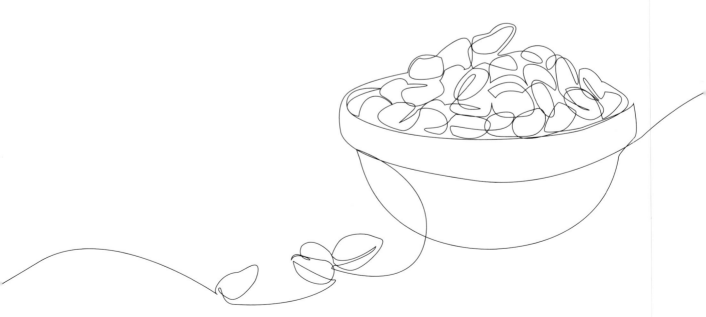

"Survival Pack" for Car, Office, or Bag

To make sticking to the any phase of the diet as easy and convenient as possible, consider keeping a supply of nonperishable foods handy in your car, desk drawer at work, or a bag. Having a "survival pack" means you're never caught in a circumstance in which you feel there's absolutely nothing appropriate for you to eat so you opt for a high-carb meal because you have no other options. With just a little planning, you'll be prepared for any situation. Here are some suggestions:

- Pouched or canned tuna, salmon, sardines, mackerel.
- Beef jerky or meat-based snack bars; always read labels and look for those that are low in carbs because some contain dried fruit and have a surprisingly high amount of total carbohydrate.
- Shelf-stable cured meats (read the package to see if they need to be refrigerated after opening).
- Pork rinds.
- Cheese crisps.
- Leakproof container of olive oil, avocado oil, or coconut oil.
- Nuts or nut butters (for Phase 2 or 3).
- Utensils and supplies: plastic silverware, napkins, paper plates, a can opener, a couple of small plastic storage containers or zip-top bags to hold leftovers or contain trash until you're able to throw it away.

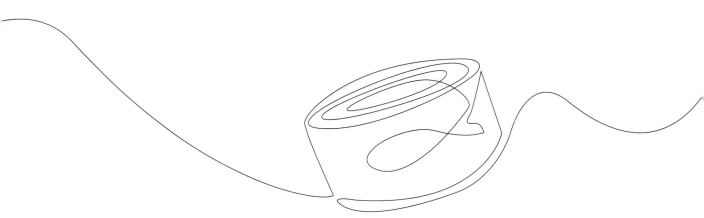

FINDING MEDICAL CARE

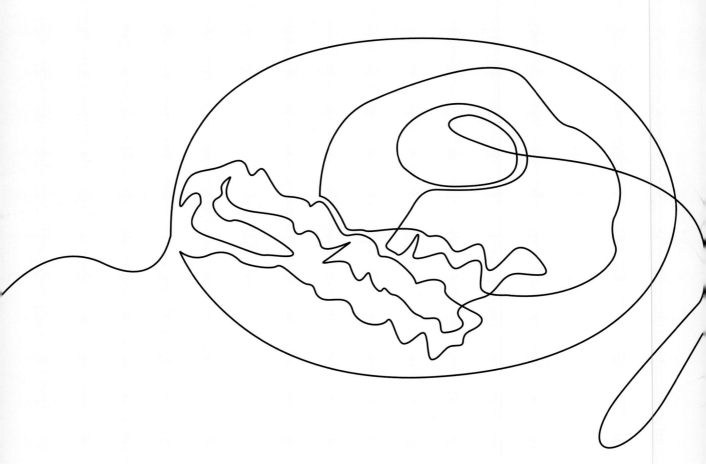

The medical and nutrition professions are gradually acknowledging that many people are consuming too much carbohydrate and that red meat, bacon, butter, egg yolks—fat and cholesterol in general—are not harmful for cardiovascular health. Changing these long-held beliefs is a slow process, though, and it may be some years before the nutritional approaches laid out by the ADAPT Your Life Diet and similar programs are accepted as a routine or standard strategy.

With that in mind, you may want to find a medical professional who is knowledgeable about ketogenic and controlled-carb diets, who'll be able to advise you in adjusting your medications if necessary, help you troubleshoot if you encounter hiccups with the diet, and interpret your bloodwork and other lab tests in the context of a low-carbohydrate hormonal milieu.

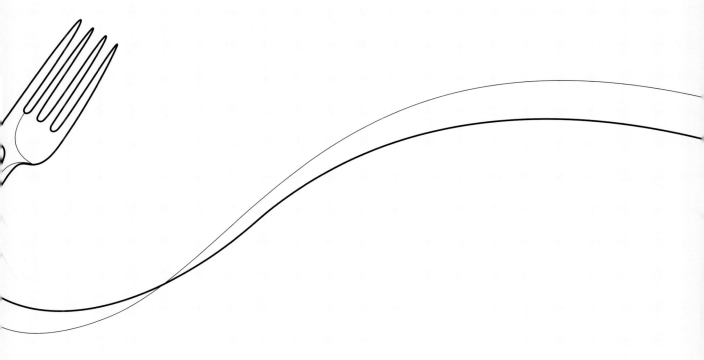

The following list includes some resources where you may be able to find a professional in your area. If you don't find anyone in your area, consider that it may well be worth a long drive, or perhaps even the cost of a plane ticket, to see a physician who's knowledgeable about the metabolic effects of the nutritional strategy you're following. Also, some of the physicians you'll see listed on these sites work remotely, and you might be able to conduct an appointment entirely by phone or online. So don't be discouraged if you don't see anyone in your immediate area. There are other ways to work with these qualified professionals.

- Ketogenic Docs: www.ketogenicdocs.com/
- Ketogenic.com doctor locator: ketogenic.com/doctors/
- Low Carb USA listing of low-carb medical practitioners: lowcarbusa.org/low-carb-providers/lchf-doctors/
- DietDoctor.com international list of low-carb doctors: dietdoctor.com/low-carb/doctors
- Obesity medicine specialists: obesitymedicine.org/find-obesity-treatment/ (Note: Not all physicians listed here are low-carb and keto-savvy, but many are.)
- Spanish: DietDoctor.com Español – Médicos que recomiendan la alimentación baja en carbos o cetogénica: dietdoctor.com/es/low-carb/medicos
- French: Les professionnels de la santé sensibilisés au régime cétogène/LCHF: eatfat2befit.com/professionnels-de-sante-lchf

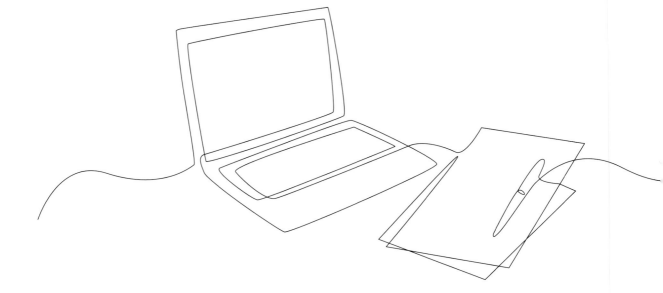

A Note About Type 1 Diabetes

Individuals with type 1 diabetes can follow ketogenic or low-carb diets, but it is critically important that you work with a medical professional who can advise you in adjusting your insulin doses. It might surprise you to learn that not only can people with type 1 diabetes follow a low-carb way of eating like ADAPT Your Life Phase 1 or Phase 2, but thousands have already been doing it for years, and their blood sugar control is impressive not just for people with type 1 diabetes, but for anyone.

As I explained in Chapter 7, there continues to be a lot of confusion in the medical and dietetics professions regarding the difference between benign nutritional ketosis and diabetic ketoacidosis. They are quite different things, and it is long past time to remove the stigma against people with type 1 diabetes implementing a dietary strategy that can greatly improve their glycemic control and overall quality of life.

If you have type 1 diabetes or know someone who does, then you know it is extremely difficult to match mealtime insulin boluses to the precise amount of carbohydrate and protein in a meal. Even when insulin is properly matched to the food, multiple variables affect sensitivity to insulin—that is, how the body reacts to insulin. Sleep quality and quantity, stress levels, exercise, illness, and numerous other factors affect insulin sensitivity daily, so maintaining healthy blood sugar levels when you have type 1 diabetes is like walking a tightrope, except it's as if two people are standing at either end of the tightrope, and each is constantly yanking it unpredictably in different directions.

It's not unusual for someone with type 1 diabetes to see blood sugar levels ranging from as low as 40 mg/dL up to 300 mg/dL (2.2 to 16.7 mmol/L) or even higher, *all in one day*. In fact, this kind of volatility—wild ups and downs in blood sugar—is fairly common in people living with this condition. This result is mainly from consuming a high-carbohydrate diet and trying to "cover" the carbs with insulin. Consuming a low-carb diet is a completely different ballgame.

When someone with type 1 diabetes eliminates the vast majority of carbo-hydrates from their diet, they need a much smaller dose of insulin to cover their protein and the minimal amount of carbs they choose to include. Using less insulin also greatly reduces the volatility in blood sugar levels. Richard Bernstein, MD, a physician managing his own type 1 diabetes with a ketogenic diet, calls this the "law of small numbers." The lower the doses of insulin you require, the lower the chances that you will experience dramatic highs and lows in blood sugar.

"The lower the doses of insulin you require, the lower the chances you'll experience **dramatic highs and lows in blood sugar.** Having type 1 diabetes is not within your control, but the added complications that may **come from using steadily increasing doses of insulin** *are.* The way to control them is to **use less insulin,** and the way to use less insulin is to **consume less carbohydrate.**

To be clear, people with type 1 diabetes will *always* need to use some insulin. Always. People with type 2 diabetes using insulin to control blood sugar may be able to discontinue their insulin injections (with physician supervision, of course) if they manage their blood sugar well enough through diet or a combination of diet and oral medications. The same is not true for people with type 1 diabetes because the two conditions are very different. However, when people with type 1 diabetes adopt a very-low-carb diet, like ADAPT Your Life Phase 1 or Phase 2, they're typically able to reduce the amount of insulin they require not just before meals but their basal bolus, too. (The basal bolus is the long-acting amount they take every day to mimic the small amount the pancreas would normally produce in a slow, steady trickle if they didn't have type 1 diabetes.)

Reducing the amount of insulin needed is beneficial because, believe it or not, people with type 1 diabetes are not immune to insulin resistance, metabolic syndrome, and all the associated issues, like cardiovascular disease, hypertension, obesity, and fatty liver. It's true—people whose bodies don't even *make* insulin can suffer the long-term consequences of having too *much* insulin! Eating a high-carb diet necessarily requires a high amount of insulin. When someone with type 1 diabetes has been using high doses of insulin for many years, they may start showing some of the same signs and symptoms of chronically high insulin that other people experience. Their bodies have become desensitized to the injected insulin, which means they require higher and higher doses to get the same blood sugar–lowering effect, the same way the pancreas in someone with type 2 diabetes or even someone who doesn't have diabetes but who has insulin resistance must secrete ever-higher amounts of insulin to keep pace with blood sugar. Insulin resistance in someone with type 1 diabetes is called "double diabetes." They had type 1 diabetes to start with, and then they developed some of the signs and symptoms of type 2 diabetes as a result of using high doses of insulin for a prolonged period. Having type 1 diabetes is not within someone's control, but the added complications that may come from using steadily increasing doses of insulin *are.* The way to control them is to use less insulin, and the way to use less insulin is to consume less carbohydrate.

Let me reiterate the importance of working with a qualified medical professional when switching to a low-carb or ketogenic diet if you have type 1 diabetes. This is nonnegotiable. You must be educated in how to adjust your insulin safely, so find a qualified professional *before* you switch your diet. Do not do this without medical supervision.

The best resources for people with type 1 diabetes who would like to follow a ketogenic or low-carb diet come from physicians who live with this condition and manage it well via carbohydrate restriction. The following books may be helpful:

- *Dr. Bernstein's Diabetes Solution* by Richard K. Bernstein, MD (also recommended are the videos from Dr. Bernstein's "Diabetes University," which you can find at www.youtube.com)

- *The Ketogenic Diet for Type 1 Diabetes* by Ellen Davis, MS, and Keith Runyan, MD

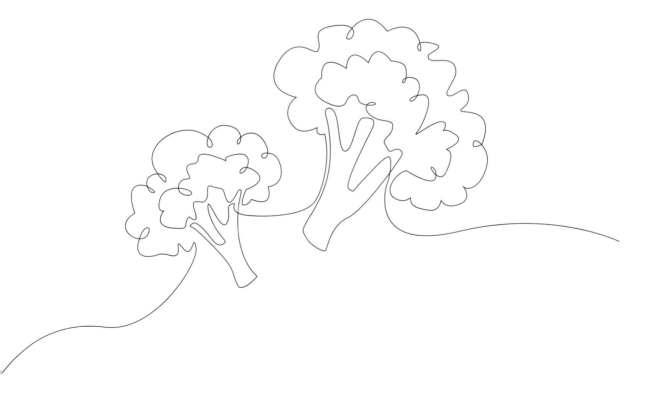

ADAPT YOUR LIFE

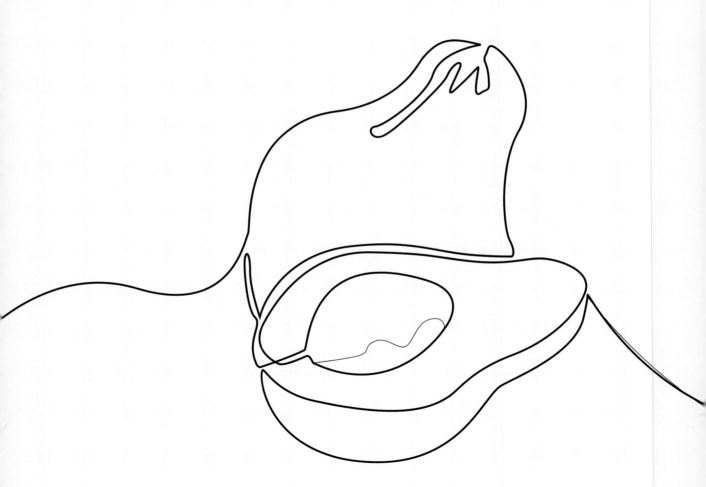

ADAPT Your Life was founded by a team of passionate health enthusiasts on a mission to inspire you to live a healthy life through a carbohydrate-aware way of eating. We knew when we started that very-low-carb ketogenic diets are extremely therapeutic and can help resolve some chronic health issues that many people have come to accept as inevitable. We've been led to believe that these conditions are normal parts of aging or that they're baked into human DNA, and people are genetically programmed to deteriorate and feel less than our best. The many thousands of people worldwide who have used low-carb and ketogenic approaches to completely transform their health and regain vitality show us that no one is destined to be unwell, and carbohydrate restriction is the solution for many who find themselves far down that path.

But we also knew that keto is only one way to be healthy, and not everyone needs to cut their carb intake by that degree. After having our own personal health transformations thanks to reduced-carb living (see Glen F.'s story on pages 162 to 163), we wanted to make it simpler and easier for others to adopt this approach. We were disappointed by the staggering amounts of sugar and other unwanted ingredients in products marketed as being wholesome or nutritious. Because we couldn't find many that we trusted and that fit the description of being low in sugar and moderate in total carbs, we started making our own, and ADAPT Your Life was born.

Our immediate mission is to bring you tasty low-carb snacks to help you live and sustain a healthy lifestyle. In the long term, our mission is much more ambitious. We are spreading awareness about controlled-carb eating through education and hands-on support via in-person workshops and online courses. To learn more about our products and our education services, visit www.adaptyourlife.com.

ADAPT Nutrition

The products we manufacture help make a no-sugar, lower-carb way of eating more convenient and *more delicious* to stay with for the long term. We have keto-friendly options as well as items more suitable to a higher carb intake. All our products are designed to minimize the impact on insulin and to help curb sugar cravings. Quality and authenticity are principles we live by—after all, we don't just make these products; we eat them, and so do our families!

Product availability is subject to change, but all our products will always be suitable for anyone limiting their sugar intake; select items will be appropriate for ketogenic diets. As of this writing, our lineup consists of the following:

Keto Bar Minis: These small morsels satisfy a craving for something sweet or crunchy with only 2-3 grams total carbs, and they're suitable for all three phases of the ADAPT Your Life Diet.

Nut + Seed Bars: These bars, which are suitable for the higher-carb end of Phase 2 and Phase 3 are chock-full of healthy fats from nuts and seeds, sweetness from erythritol, and a healthy dose of fiber.

Protein Bars: Packed with protein from collagen and whey, healthy fats from MCT oil and palm oil, and a generous amount of fiber, these bars are a great snack between meals, while traveling, or before a workout when you're on the higher-carb end of Phase 2 or in Phase 3.

ADAPT Education and Events

Dr. Westman has spent more than two decades conducting and publishing research establishing the beneficial impact of ketogenic and low-carb diets across an array of health issues, including type 2 diabetes, obesity, PCOS, GERD, and more. Through the online seminars and traveling events, we hope to help grow and support low-carb communities around the world.

ADAPT Your Life Academy

End Your Carb Confusion was written with the intention that anyone reading it would be able to identify their carbohydrate tolerance and construct a diet to help them reach optimal health. Additional support, education, and encouragement can only help, though, and you can find that support in our online courses and seminars (www.adaptyourlifeacademy.com). If you're not quite sure if or when it's time to try transitioning to a different phase of the diet, or if you need help with the everyday nuts and bolts of implementing the diet and sticking with it—suggestions for what to buy at the grocery store, for example, or tips on how to put simple meals together—the online courses are your source for extra guidance that can make it simpler and easier to reap the benefits of lower-carb living for a lifetime. Seem to be doing everything right but not getting your desired results? We've got you covered with troubleshooting common issues. Courses also take a closer look at individual medical concerns for people who want a deeper understanding of the root causes of metabolic illness and explain why using the ADAPT Your Life Diet framework to control blood sugar, insulin, and inflammation is effective for resolving so many of them.

Events

ADAPT Events are one-day seminars during which Dr. Westman and keto- and low-carb-savvy medical and nutrition professionals from the local area educate and support local communities regarding the scientifically supported therapeutic benefits of a low-sugar, controlled-carbohydrate lifestyle. Community members also share testimonials about their success using lower-carb nutrition to reclaim their health. Whether you're brand-new to low-carb eating or you feel like a seasoned pro, ADAPT Events are a way to connect "in real life" with people in your community who are following a similar path.

If you're having a difficult time living without sweet and starchy favorites from your former high-carb life, attending an event can reinspire and reinvigorate you. Events include a Q&A session, so you can get help from the professionals for troubleshooting your diet, and Dr. Westman delivers a workshop to reinforce the simple basics of the ADAPT framework.

Educational Videos

ADAPT Your Life is honored to feature doctors, nurses, nutritionists, dietitians, researchers, personal trainers, and other allied health and fitness professionals on our YouTube channel (channel name: ADAPT Your Life). There we provide thousands of hours of education on starting and staying with ketogenic or controlled-carb diets—completely free and at your fingertips. If you can't make it to an event, our videos are the next best thing, and even if you do come to an event, our videos give you instant access to trustworthy information any time you want it. Videos also feature success stories from people whose lives have been transformed by this simple change in diet, much like the success stories shared in this book.

FOOD LISTS FOR PHASE 1, PHASE 2, AND PHASE 3

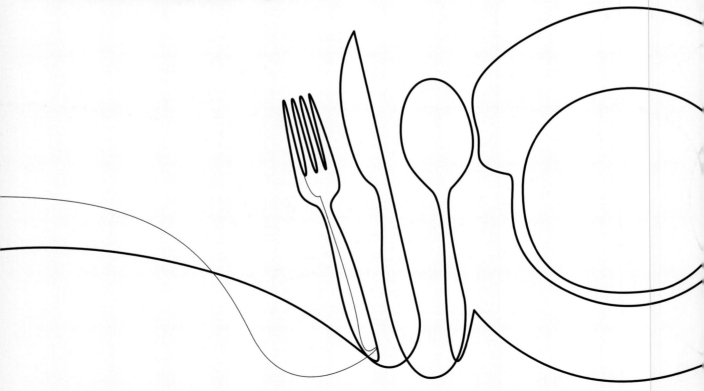

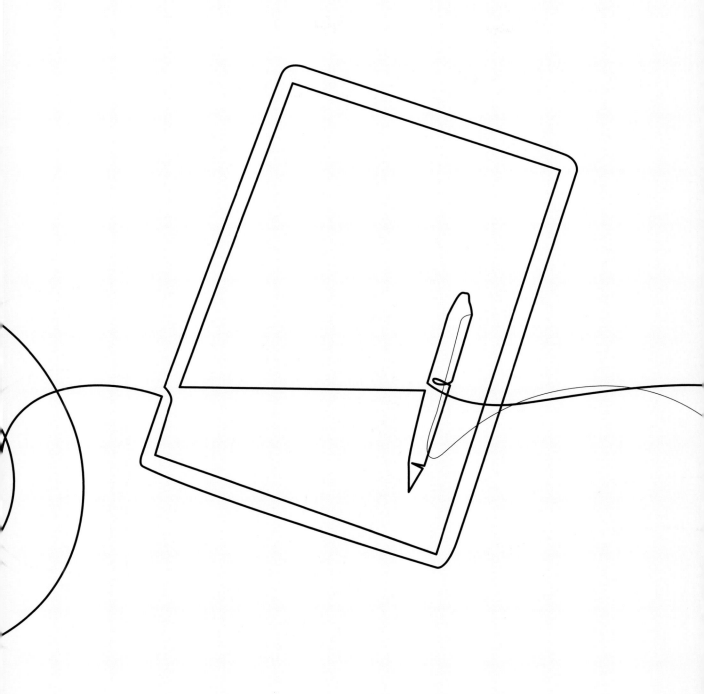

ADAPT Your Life Phase 1 Food List

Food type	How much	What
Proteins	All you like until comfortably full but not stuffed	Beef, pork, lamb, bison, venison, chicken, turkey, duck, eggs (includes yolks), finfish, shellfish (except oysters and clams), other animal proteins (game meats)
Salad vegetables	Up to 2 cups per day (measured uncooked)	Arugula, bok choy, cabbage (all varieties), chard, chives, endive, greens (beet, collard, mustard, and turnip greens), kale, lettuce (all varieties), parsley, radicchio, radishes, scallions, spinach, watercress
Nonstarchy vegetables	Up to 1 cup per day (measured uncooked)	Artichokes, asparagus, broccoli, Brussels sprouts, cauliflower, celery, celery root (celeriac), cucumber, eggplant (aubergine), fennel, green beans (string beans), jicama, kohlrabi, leeks, mushrooms, okra, onions, bell peppers (capsicum), other peppers (poblano, serrano, jalapeño, etc.), unsweetened pumpkin, rhubarb, shallots, snow peas, sprouts (bean and alfalfa), sugar-snap peas, summer squash, tomatoes, wax beans, zucchini (courgette)
Cheese	Up to 4 ounces per day	• Any hard, aged cheese: Asiago, blue, brie, Camembert, cheddar, Colby, Emmental, Gouda, Gruyère, mozzarella, Parmesan, provolone, Swiss, etc. • Soft fresh cheeses (goat cheese, cream cheese): check label for carb count
Added fats and oils	2-tablespoon maximum per day of each	• Mayonnaise • Butter, ghee, oils, heavy cream, sour cream • Oil-based salad dressings
Limited quantity foods	Maximums per day	• Soy sauce: 2 tablespoons • Lemon or lime juice: 2 tablespoons • Avocado: ½ fruit • Pickles: 2 servings • Olives: 6
Condiments	Read labels to stay under 20 total carbs per day for all your food	Mustard, vinegar (go easy on balsamic), unsweetened hot sauce, salsa, low-carb salad dressings (watch the total fat), fresh or dried herbs and spices
Zero-carb snacks	Unlimited within reason	Pork rinds, sugar-free fruit-flavored gelatin, pepperoni or salami slices, hard-boiled eggs, zero-sugar beef jerky
Fruit	None	—
Nuts and seeds	None	—
Beverages	Unlimited	Water, tea (hot or iced—no sugar), coffee (watch the amount of cream), sugar-free or unsweetened flavored drinks, diet soda, unsweetened flavored seltzer/sparkling water

Notes:

- The amounts listed are maximums to stay under, not minimums to aim for every day.

- These are the foods that are *permitted*, not that are *required*. You do not need to eat 2 cups of leafy greens and 1 cup of nonstarchy vegetables per day if you do not want to. You do not need to use added fats and oils if you are satisfied with the fat that comes naturally with your meat, poultry, cheese, and so on.

- Proteins: All cuts are permitted—chops, roasts, steaks, ground meats, sausage (no sugar or starchy fillers), bacon, cured or processed meats (salami, pepperoni, lunchmeat—read labels for total carbs), all poultry cuts, organ meats.

- Seafood: Canned fish is permitted (tuna, salmon, sardines, mackerel); avoid imitation seafood.

- If you are trying to lose body fat, use added fats and oils sparingly. Enjoy the fat that occurs naturally in meat, eggs, seafood, poultry, and cheese. If you are living with a health problem but are not carrying excess body weight, you may consume larger quantities of fats and oils.

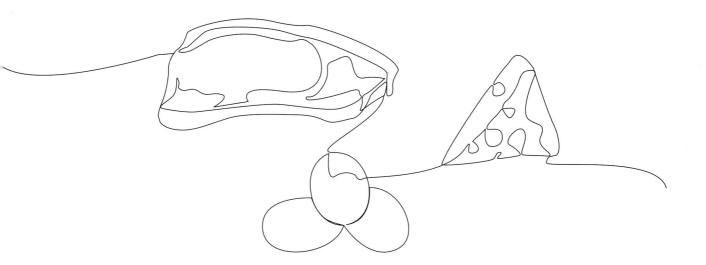

ADAPT Your Life Phase 2 Food List

Food type	How much	What
Proteins	All you like until comfortably full but not stuffed	Beef, pork, lamb, bison, venison, chicken, turkey, duck, eggs (includes yolks), finfish, shellfish (except oysters and clams), other animal proteins (game meats)
Salad vegetables	4 cups per day (measured uncooked)	Arugula, bok choy, cabbage (all varieties), chard, chives, endive, greens (beet, collard, mustard, and turnip greens), kale, lettuce (all varieties), parsley, radicchio, radishes, scallions, spinach, watercress
Nonstarchy vegetables + Phase 2 vegetables	2 cups per day of nonstarchy veg OR 1 cup per day nonstarchy veg plus 1 cup per day Phase 2 vegetables (measured uncooked)	• Nonstarchy: Artichokes, asparagus, broccoli, Brussels sprouts, cauliflower, celery, celery root (celeriac), cucumber (includes nonsweet pickles), eggplant (aubergine), fennel, green beans (string beans), jicama, kohlrabi, leeks, mushrooms, okra, onions, peppers (bell, poblano, serrano, jalapeño, etc.), unsweetened pumpkin, rhubarb, shallots, snow peas, sprouts (bean and alfalfa), sugar-snap peas, summer squash, tomatoes, wax beans, zucchini (courgette) • Phase 2 vegetables: Beets, carrots, rutabaga, turnips, winter squash (acorn, butternut, hubbard, spaghetti)
Cheese	4 ounces per day	All cheeses—aged, fresh, soft, hard (read labels for carb count in processed cheese products)
Added fats and oils	Maximums per day	• Mayonnaise: 2 tablespoons • Butter, ghee, oils, heavy cream, sour cream: 3 tablespoons • Oil-based salad dressings: 2 tablespoons
Limited quantity foods	Maximums per day	• Soy sauce: 3 tablespoons • Avocado: 1 fruit • Olives: 12
Condiments	See note*	Mustard, vinegar (go easy on balsamic), unsweetened hot sauce, salsa, sugar-free ketchup, low-carb salad dressings (watch the total fat), lemon/lime juice, fresh or dried herbs and spices
Zero-carb snacks	Unlimited within reason	Pork rinds, sugar-free fruit-flavored gelatin, pepperoni or salami slices, hard-boiled eggs, zero-sugar beef jerky
Fruit	½ cup berries or 1 small to medium fruit per day	Apricots, blackberries, blueberries, cranberries (fresh and unsweetened, not dried), nectarines, peaches, plums, raspberries, strawberries,
Nuts and seeds	2 ounces per day	All nuts and seeds (go easy on higher-carb items: peanuts, cashews, pistachios)
Dairy	Maximums per day*	• Plain, unsweetened yogurt or sugar-free flavored yogurt: 1 cup • Cottage cheese: 1 cup • Ricotta cheese: ½ cup
Low-carb grain products	See note*	Low carb, high-fiber crispbreads, crackers, wraps, flatbreads

Keep your portions to sizes that allow you to stay under 50 grams of total carbs per day for all your food.

Notes:

- The amounts listed are maximums to stay under, not minimums to aim for every day.

- These are the foods that are permitted, not that are required. You do not need to eat 3 cups of leafy greens and 2 cups of nonstarchy vegetables per day if you do not want to. You do not need to use added fats and oils if you are satisfied with the fat that comes naturally with your meat, poultry, cheese, and so on.

- Proteins: All cuts are permitted—chops, roasts, steaks, ground meats, sausage (no sugar), bacon, cured or processed meats (salami, pepperoni, lunchmeat—read labels for total carbs), all poultry cuts, organ meats.

- Seafood: Canned fish is permitted (tuna, salmon, sardines, mackerel); avoid imitation seafood.

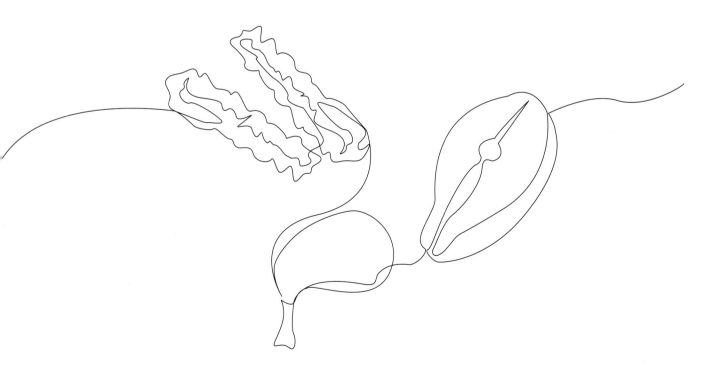

ADAPT Your Life Phase 3 Food List

Food type	How much	What
Proteins	All you like until comfortably full but not stuffed	*Beef, pork, lamb, bison, venison, chicken, turkey, duck, eggs (includes yolks), finfish, shellfish, other animal proteins (game meats)*
Salad vegetables	Unlimited*	*Arugula, bok choy, cabbage (all varieties), chard, chives, endive, greens (beet, collard, mustard, and turnip greens), kale, lettuce (all varieties), parsley, radicchio, radishes, scallions, spinach, watercress*
Other vegetables	Unlimited*	*Artichokes, asparagus, avocado, beets, broccoli, Brussels sprouts, carrots, cauliflower, celery, celery root (celeriac), cucumber, eggplant (aubergine), fennel, green beans (string beans), jicama, kohlrabi, leeks, mushrooms, okra, olives, onions, parsnips, peppers (bell, poblano, serrano, jalapeño, etc.), pumpkin, rhubarb, rutabaga, shallots, snow peas, sprouts (bean and alfalfa), sugar-snap peas, summer squash, tomatoes, turnips, wax beans, winter squash (acorn, butternut, hubbard, spaghetti), zucchini (courgette)*
Starchy root vegetables	1 medium to large per day or 1-serving equivalent	*Sweet potatoes, white potatoes, yams, yuca/cassava*
Cheese and other dairy	Use high-fat dairy sparingly if weight is a concern	• *All cheeses—aged, fresh, soft, hard: 5 ounces* • *Unsweetened or sugar-free flavored yogurt: 1 to 2 cups* • *Cottage cheese: 1 to 2 cups*
Added fats and oils	Maximums per day (Use less if weight is a concern)	• *Mayonnaise: 3 tablespoons* • *Butter, ghee, oils, heavy cream, sour cream: 4 tablespoons* • *Oil-based salad dressings: 4 tablespoons*
Condiments	See note*	*Mustard, vinegar, unsweetened hot sauce, salsa, salad dressings, lemon/lime juice, sugar-free ketchup, fresh or dried herbs and spices*
Zero-carb snacks	Unlimited within reason	*Pork rinds, sugar-free fruit-flavored gelatin, pepperoni or salami slices, hard-boiled eggs, zero-sugar beef jerky*
Fruit	See note*	*All fruits (favor fresh, whole fruit over canned or dried)*
Nuts and seeds	4 ounces per day	*All nuts and seeds*
Beans, legumes, pulses	1 to 2 cups*	*All beans, legumes, and pulses: black beans, edamame, garbanzos, green peas, lentils, lima, kidney, navy, turtle, etc.*
Grains	1 to 2 cups*	*Amaranth, barley, buckwheat, corn, millet, oats, quinoa, rice, spelt, wheat, other grains*

Keep your portions to sizes that allow you to stay under 150 grams of total carbs per day for all your food.

Notes:

- No foods are off-limits for Phase 3 except sugar. Keep your total carbohydrate intake for the day to 150 grams or less. Consume more carbs on hard training days if needed.

- The amounts listed are maximums to stay under, not minimums to aim for every day.

- These are the foods that are permitted, not that are required. You do not need to eat large amounts of vegetables or to consume starchy vegetables, beans, or grains if you do not want to. You do not need use a lot of added fats and oils if you are satisfied with the fat that comes naturally with your meat, poultry, eggs, cheese, etc.

- Proteins: All cuts are permitted—chops, roasts, steaks, ground meats, sausage (no sugar), bacon, cured or processed meats (salami, pepperoni, lunchmeat—read labels for total carbs), all poultry cuts, organ meats

- Seafood: Canned fish is permitted (tuna, salmon, sardines, mackerel)

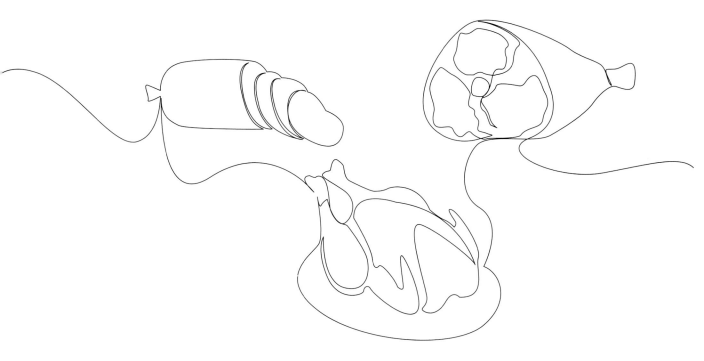

ACKNOWLEDGMENTS

There are two author names on the cover of this book, but don't let that fool you. The education and experience that have allowed us to write this book didn't occur in a vacuum. We are both indebted to numerous individuals who have served as mentors, colleagues, and teachers, and whose wisdom and guidance have helped shape our careers and our personal health journeys.

Several names immediately come to mind. These intrepid researchers and clinicians possessed the bravery and scientific integrity to go against the grain—literally and figuratively—at a time when questioning the validity of longstanding mainstream recommendations to limit intake of foods high in saturated fat or cholesterol was grounds for near-excommunication from professional organizations and made for the quick disappearance of funding for research. The contributions of Steve Phinney, MD, PhD; Jeff Volek, PhD, RD; Michael Eades, MD; Mary Dan Eades, MD; Richard Feinman, PhD; Richard K. Bernstein, MD; Ron Rosedale, MD; William Yancy Jr., MD; and others too numerous to mention by name built the foundation upon which current research is built—much of which these individuals continue to spearhead. This foundation, in turn, was built upon earlier work by George Cahill, Richard Veech, and other scientists who elucidated biochemical and physiological mechanisms regarding ketones and ketogenesis.

Two doctors merit special recognition, as they faced legal action or professional censure for daring to suggest that decreasing the amount of carbohydrate in one's diet is safe and might have beneficial effects for health. To Timothy "Prof" Noakes, MD, and Gary Fettke, MD, we and the rest of the low-carb community can only hope that the emotional tolls of the profound burdens you and your loved ones faced and the prolonged disruptions inflicted upon your professional and personal lives are lessened through knowing that the international attention your situations garnered introduced countless more people to carbohydrate restriction and the myriad improvements it facilitates in health and quality of life.

We also owe a debt of gratitude to the patients we've treated and the clients we've worked with. Your experiences with ketogenic and low-carb diets have taught us as much, if not more, than textbooks and published papers. Understanding physiology and biochemical mechanisms is critical, but it's equally important to understand how to translate these into commonsense advice people can put into practice in the real world. In fact, patients serving as teachers are what changed the course of Dr. Westman's career from general internal medicine to keto medicine and specializing in obesity and type 2 diabetes. His curiosity was piqued over two decades ago when two patients at the Veterans Affairs Medical Center in Durham, North Carolina, lost substantial amounts of weight and showed impressive improvements in measurements related to blood sugar and cardiovascular health by following a low-carb diet—the Atkins diet, to be specific.

Professionals outside the medical and nutrition professions have also shone light upon the questionable origins of advice to limit intake of foods rich in saturated fat and cholesterol while emphasizing complex carbohydrates as the base of a healthy diet. Journalists Nina Teicholz (author of *The Big Fat Surprise*) and Gary Taubes (author of *Good Calories, Bad Calories* and *The Case for Keto*), along with nurse Belinda Fettke, have been instrumental in exposing the politics, religious influence, and vested economic interests that overshadowed and continue to overshadow the science regarding population-wide dietary recommendations. This work is every bit as critical to educating people as are face-to-face visits with physicians.

Equally important are the efforts of laypeople who share their remarkable low-carb transformations and provide support and advice for others. There's a gulf between knowing what to do and actually doing it. These individuals help bridge that gulf through recipes, encouragement, education, tough love, camaraderie, and, above all, empathy and understanding. Social media abounds with such transformations and big-hearted people, but a few deserve special mention for the roles they have played in our professional and personal lives. To Casey Durango, Tyler Cartwright, Kristie Sullivan, Jimmy Moore, RD Dikeman, Carl Franklin, Richard Morris, Glen and Yael Finkel, Liza Becker, Doug Reynolds, Pam Devine, and the many we are no doubt forgetting, *thank you.* Jenny Gough Short belongs on this list but also deserves individual distinction for providing some of the illustrations in this book. Your artwork brings our book to life, Jenny. Thank you for sharing your talent with us and our readers.

Although certain potential applications of low-carb and ketogenic diets are beyond the scope of this book, we would like to acknowledge the exciting work being done by researchers and clinicians whose expertise is outside the realm of weight loss, type 2 diabetes, and metabolic syndrome. Although still in its early days, emerging research suggests ketones and/or ketogenic diets may have therapeutic potential for rare or difficult-to-treat conditions, such as glycogen storage diseases, cerebral palsy, lipedema, lymphedema, migraine, Alzheimer's disease, Parkinson's disease, and psychiatric conditions including schizophrenia, bipolar disorder, and depression. A burgeoning field called *metabolic psychiatry* may hold promise for millions of people living with intractable and medication-refractory mental illnesses.

Finally, to the late Robert C. Atkins, MD, and Jackie Eberstein, RN, his long-time partner at the Atkins Center for Complementary Medicine: Dr. Atkins, you were right: You did not live to see your implicitly successful method of carbohydrate restriction be formally scientifically validated and accepted more broadly among medical professionals, but Jackie and your beloved Veronica are witnessing this before their eyes. They continue to carry your message, educating a new generation of medical and nutrition professionals and patients alike about the life-changing effects of a simple dietary change. Jackie and Veronica, may we all follow your lead and continue to honor Dr. Atkins' legacy of helping people restore their health and improve their lives through eating delicious food.

INDEX

muscle cramps, during Phase 1, 119
mustard, in Phase 1, 75

N

natural sugar, 45
natural sweeteners, 186
nerve damage, blood sugar and, 24
net carbs, 59
neuropathy, blood sugar and, 24
noodles, substitutions for, 76
Nut + Seed Bars (ADAPT Your Life), 220
nutrients, sugar and, 21–22
nutrition facts label, 177–179
nutritional ketosis, 88, 91–92
nutritional supplements, 153–155
nuts
   in Phase 1, 95
   in Phase 2, 127, 132

O

obesity
   growth of, 12–13
   personal stories about, 40–41, 66–69, 136–139, 188–191
obesity medicine specialists (website), 214
oils, in Phase 1, 74
olives, on Phase 1, 74
online seminars (ADAPT), 220–221
organic, 187
overtraining, in Phase 3, 155–157

P

Pakistani cuisine, 207
pasture-raised, 187
PCOS, 35–36, 40–41

performance decline, as a symptom of overtraining, 156
personal stories
   April K., 200–203
   Cheryl B., 66–69
   Gayle H., 122–123
   Glen F., 162–163
   Jeff C., 188–191
   Kim C., 48–49
   Larry D., 136–139
   Rachel G., 40–41
   Robyn D., 28–29
   Sandra W., 174–175
personality changes, as a symptom of overtraining, 156
Phase 1 of ADAPT Your Life Diet
   about, 71–72
   benefits of, 112–113
   difference in, 77–78
   emotion-based eating, 78
   FAQ, 80–111
   fat loss during, 113–115
   food lists for, 73–76, 224–225
   gallbladders and, 180
   getting started on, 79
   meal/snack ideas for, 195–196
   priorities during, 115–117
   resources for, 121
   sample menus for, 77
   special considerations for, 118–120
   transitioning to Phase 2 from, 121
Phase 2 of ADAPT Your Life Diet
   about, 125–126, 134–135
   food lists for, 127–128, 226–227
   gallbladders and, 180
   meal/snack ideas for, 196
   preparing for Phase 3, 135–137
   sample menus, 129
   tips for success with, 130–131
   transitioning from Phase 1 to, 121, 131–134